The Parent-Child Dance

The Parent-Child Dance

Strategies and Techniques for Staying One Step Ahead

Ronald A. Kotkin, PhD
Professor Emeritus
University of California, Irvine

Aubrey H. Fine, EdD
Professor
California State Polytechnic University, Pomona

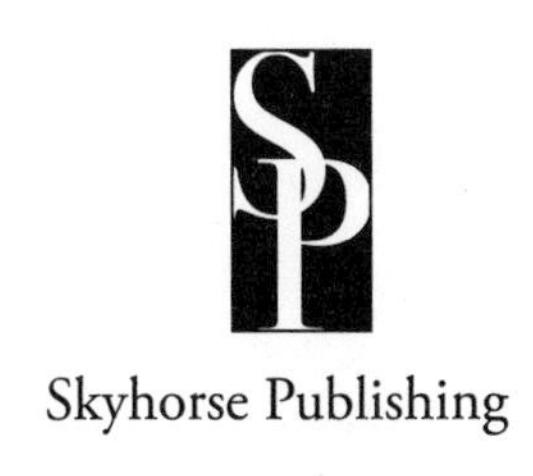

Skyhorse Publishing

Skyhorse Publishing books may be purchased in bulk at special discounts for sales promotion, corporate gifts, fund-raising, or educational purposes. Special editions can also be created to specifications. For details, contact the Special Sales Department, Skyhorse Publishing, 307 West 36th Street, 11th Floor, New York, NY 10018 or info@skyhorsepublishing.com.

Skyhorse® and Skyhorse Publishing® are registered trademarks of Skyhorse Publishing, Inc.®, a Delaware corporation.

Visit our website at www.skyhorsepublishing.com.

10 9 8 7 6 5 4 3 2 1

Library of Congress Cataloging-in-Publication Data is available on file.

Cover design by Laura Klynstra

Print ISBN: 978-1-63220-294-9
Ebook ISBN: 978-1-63220-882-8

Printed in the United States of America

Contents

Dedication VII

Acknowledgements VIII

Foreword IX

An Invitation to the Parent-Child Dance XII

SECTION I 1

Chapter 1: The Journey Begins with Taking the First Step 3

SECTION II 25

Introduction to Section II 27

Chapter 2: Learning Basic Steps: Understanding Techniques That Make Leading Easier 29

Chapter 3: Motivating the Dancers 51

Chapter 4: No Time for Tap Dancing—Let's Tango: Steps to Decrease Non-Compliance and Opposition 78

Chapter 5: Avoiding Missteps 101

Chapter 6: Helping Your Child Make Friends 123

SECTION III 149

Chapter 7: *Transitions in the Dance Steps: Tweaking for the Pre-Teen and Teen Years* 151

Chapter 8: *Enhancing Life within the Family: Recipes to Make Home Life More Meaningful and Enjoyable* 182

Chapter 9: *The Family That Plays Together Stays Together: Enriching Our Families with Leisure, Sports, and Companion Animals* 199

Chapter 10: *Pointing Your Child to a Life of Resiliency: A Lifetime Journey* 221

Dedication

Ron

I dedicate this book to "Ret" whose love, support, patience, and feedback helped me to complete this book. I also dedicate this book to Carlos, Erin, and their incredible daughter, Ellie. Their commitment to Ellie is what this book is about.

Aubrey

I dedicate this book to my wife and partner, Nya, who has blessed my life for close to forty years. You have made parenting together a true joy.

I also dedicate this book to my boys, Sean and Corey, who have allowed me to feel and live the true essence of being a Dad. You have made me realize how lucky I am to have had this life experience.

Finally I dedicate this book to all the parents who I have had the pleasure to work with over the years. I am honored to have been of support to you and your children.

Acknowledgements

Borrowing from the phrase "It takes a village to raise a child," this book would not have come to fruition without the help and support of many. The following are several people that we would like to recognize and thank.

We are very grateful to Alexandra Hess and Joseph Sverchek and the staff at Skyhorse Publishing for stewarding this book and helping us to bring it to completion.

We are indebted to the following people for their support in gathering some of the research for this book that we utilized: Julia Gimeno, Joanna Cole, Katie Weimerslage, Laurie Bailon, Christine Delman, Melissa Bladh, and Alexandria Martinez.

The authors would like to thank Krista Trapani for her efforts in graphically designing the Backpack of Resilience in Chapter 10. We would also like to thank Clara Kramer for her help in suggesting a graphic design for the cover of the book. We truly appreciated your professionalism and creativity. Over the course of the past year, several people read earlier drafts of the various chapters and provided input and editorial comments. We are sincerely indebted to all of these individuals for their suggestions:

Rudi Gomez, Stephen Davis, Dale Salwak, Charles R. Kotkin, Christine Bowers, Clara Cramer, Julia Gimeno, Teal Mackintosh, Pam Seggerman, John Ugaldie, Susan Siaw, Sue Keir, John Brady, Chris Loidolt, Loretta Kotkin, Nya Fine, and Tera Bernard.

Foreword

My daughter spent the first five weeks of her life outside the womb in the NICU—the Neonatal Intensive Care Unit. She arrived almost exactly two months to the day before her due date. She was doing things *her* way, disregarding what others expected of her. My wife and I were in shock seeing her so soon, so early. My daughter was raring to go, breathing on her own, kicking back in her incubator. She was the tiniest human I'd ever seen, despite the fact that the NICU staff told us she was big for her age—a whopping four pounds. My wife and I stood on each side of the incubator, staring down at our daughter in awe. I made the formal introductions, whispering to her, "We're your parents, kid." She smiled. This wasn't my imagination. My wife saw it too. It was probably gas. Her mother is convinced she understood. It had to have been gas.

My daughter's independent streak continued in the hospital as she routinely pulled off whatever wires were connected to her, growled with annoyance at diaper changes, and otherwise let it be known when her needs or desires were not being met. When we finally brought her home, we were suddenly on our own, without a professional staff to step in and care for our daughter 24/7. As stressful as it was to visit the hospital on a daily basis, my wife and I joked that we had the best babysitters anyone could possibly ask for. And then we didn't.

Having our daughter home was wonderful, but there were growing pains. I had never spent much time around children, much less an infant—much less my own child (this was my first). My wife stayed at home for two months. As the day of her return to work neared, I genuinely wondered aloud who was going to take care of our daughter. It should not have come as a surprise, though it did, when my wife responded, "You."

I did not have a 9 to 5 job; I did my work at home and could set my own hours—which meant I was automatically bestowed the title of Stay-At-Home Dad. Suddenly, it was just me and the kid—the two of us getting to know each other. My daughter did not come with a manual. Consequently, my role as a father came with a lot of on-the-job training. Her disapproval of diaper changes continued at home. She would cry and yell and generally protest whenever I set her down on the changing table. After a while, I began to discern her cries—which ones were real and which were fake. Her cries on the changing table were *always* fake. One time, when she was putting particular gusto into her performance during a diaper change, I matter-of-factly told her, "I know you're faking it." Amazingly, she immediately stopped crying. Or perhaps not so amazingly. Maybe she realized her tactics were futile in this particular instance and decided to conserve her energy.

One thing that happens when you become a parent is you begin to spend more time with other parents and less time with your single friends who are eager to tell you about the cutest thing their dog did that day. As my wife and I visited with other friends who were parents, along with their children, we found ourselves swapping war stories. One friend told us of his seemingly angelic two-year-old son who threw a tantrum while sitting in his high chair. He simply did not want to continue eating his meal. His father attempted to strike a deal with him. "One more bite and you can get down." This did not suffice. His son began kicking and screaming at the top of his lungs. That's when his mom rushed into the room and immediately removed him from the high chair, placing him on the floor.

The boy turned to his father and with a victorious smile said, "One more bite. Get down." I've come to the conclusion that babies, toddlers, and children know everything. At least they know everything in terms of how to deal with big people. Meanwhile, the big people are often left to fumble in the dark, haplessly attempting to determine whether those cries are legitimate or downright manipulation. It's not just the crying. It's everything. Every waking moment a child is assessing how much leeway they have in any given situation. The parent-child relationship is definitely a dance. Each participant is doing their best to determine what the other's next move is going to be.

Don't get me wrong—I don't mean to sound as if children are ruthless, calculating, tactical, and opportunistic. *Of course* they are. They're also cute and cuddly and beautiful and inspiring and loving and fun and spectacular. When friends of mine come into town and I show them around Los Angeles, I get just as excited about things I've seen a thousand times as they do because they're seeing something for the first time. Having a kid is like that, only a gazillion times more intense. You're like their tour guide *of life*.

I still remember the day I showed my daughter a papaya for the first time. I held it up and told her, "This is a papaya. Your first papaya. I was here the day you saw it." She was riveted. I was excited about the papaya too! (My wife later pointed out it was a spaghetti squash, but you get the point.) Having a kid is an exhilarating ride with twists and turns and challenges beyond anticipation. If only the kid came with a manual. In those early days and not so early days, I often thought it would be helpful if there were a book that cut through the clinical mumbo jumbo and explained things in a way I could easily understand. This is that book.

Carlos Kotkin is the author of the dating memoir *Please God Let It Be Herpes: A Heartfelt Quest for Love and Companionship.* He has written humorous articles for the *New York Times, Sunset Magazine, Marie Claire* and other publications. His live storytelling performances have been featured on NPR's *The Moth Radio Hour*, KCRW's *UnFictional* and in the popular podcast *Risk!* He is one of the screenwriters of the animated feature *Rio 2.*

An Invitation to the Parent-Child Dance

You are cordially invited to a dance. Not a typical dance or an average cotillion that you may attend with your child, but a journey that will be memorable and could change your life. If you accept the invitation, you may have one or several partners going along with you. The music will only be heard in your mind as you dance the nights away. This won't be the typical dance with your son or daughter, but rather, a lifelong series of daily events of moving and interacting with your child. You will find no address for the dance. It will not be held in a formal ballroom or social hall but in your home on an ongoing basis. Have we piqued your curiosity about accepting our invitation?

The invitation is to attend a journey in life where you will not only learn to appreciate the gems in your life, but how to interact and enjoy being with one another. You will learn new dance moves, but they will not be the salsa, rumba, or waltz that you are familiar with. These dances will consist of new movements that will include planned interactions with your child that will assist in making your relationships more meaningful and unbreakable. The art of dancing and parenting can be viewed in a similar fashion because they both have to do with movement and expression. They both can be done with others. In parenting, our movements with our children can be enhanced not only by our passion and commitment, but also by learning methods that assist us in enhancing our relationships with our children.

Choreography conjures images of art. It highlights the planned steps and movements that a dancer, actor, or even a magician uses to perform a certain act. The choreography plan allows for the final fluidity and naturalness that is witnessed in the actual performance. Choreography can also be witnessed in our interactions with our children. It encompasses our planned intentions of how to best interact and parent.

The key question to ask is, how will we create an experience that helps our young children to dance with us, to express themselves in a natural way, but also to recognize that we dance together? The concept of choreography isn't only related to the techniques we apply, it also relates to the passion and commitment that we have for nurturing our children. Optimal parenting must combine viable techniques with love and commitment to our children.

The book is divided into three sections. The first section introduces the Parent-Child Dance and discusses the many facets that influence our roles. In the second section, we illustrate the choreography of the Parent-Child Dance and highlight a wide array of proven, effective approaches that encourage your child's compliance and a willingness to put out his/her best efforts. We have included the periodic inclusion of segments of dialogue often expressed during our work with families on how children and their parents may think about the changes we are proposing. These examples should be very helpful to you in understanding the proposed techniques.

Finally the third section of the book is more general and provides answers to many questions that you may have about home life issues, such as sibling rivalry, sports in your childrens' lives, their roles in the family, and conflict resolution. There are also chapters on some of the different methods of parenting teens, as well as suggestions of how we might help guide our children to a life of resilience.

Well, there you have it. We hope you will accept our invitation. You may never look at the word "choreography" or "dance" the same way now. Who would have ever thought that dancing could be so valuable to our young ones? Get your pencils ready and your dance shoes on. Let the movement and the dance of life begin!

All our best,

Ron and Aubrey

SECTION I

CHAPTER 1

The Journey Begins with Taking the First Step

There they stood, Mom in her royal blue evening gown, her firstborn son dressed to the T. All eyes were upon them as they were about to begin their ceremonial mom and son dance. The music had been selected by both of them months ago. However, the spirit of their dance had been percolating since Sean was born. Nya (Mom), was beaming with joy as she embraced Sean. She had nurtured him from birth, and now it was time to let him soar. Her boy was growing up and was beginning a new chapter in his life. They shed tears of joy moments before the music started. In silence, as all the guests watched them, what were they thinking of? Were memories of the years gone by flittering about in both their minds? Only they knew for sure. But for that moment, time seemed frozen as they waited. Although their dance was about to begin, their parent-child dance, in essence, their relationship, had begun so many years before, and today was one of their blessings from that relationship.

Parenting is a figurative dance. It is probably one of the most complicated (and ever evolving) dances we will ever have to learn. This dance involves our abilities to shift, lead, and move with our children in order to make the process appear seamless. Unlike recreational dancing, the dance we have with our children has a major impact on real life. We need to strive for excellence because the stakes are quite high. Our success in this dance will determine if we will strengthen or weaken our relationships with our children. We all need to appreciate that parenting isn't about bossing our children around, but rather teaching, and communicating with them. Strong parents learn how to lead their family through tough times so that their children will follow and do what is needed to become the most self-sufficient beings that they can be.

Before discussing the metaphor of the parent-child dance, let's return to our opening story about the wedding. In April 2011, Aubrey's firstborn got married. The event provides a lovely example with which to open this book. "I can still see both of them (the new married couple) with their eyes gazing upon each other. It is a day I will always cherish," Aubrey admitted. "I, too, had tears of joy in my eyes. Watching them allowed me to put into perspective all of the years that we had spent building up to this point." Our childrens' growth is dependent upon many influences, but for sure our parental imprint had something to do with it as well. Today they are dancing to the music of their lives, and we are witnesses to it.

On his wedding day, I celebrated somewhat differently my dance (relationship) with my son; I officiated his wedding. The ceremony itself was a remarkable experience as I was able to look into my son's eyes while he gazed longingly at his bride to be. During the ceremony, I remember sharing with both of them some inspirational advice shared by my grandfather when I was a young man. His words were inspirational, and I have always kept them close to my heart. He said, "Make a life, not a living." These same simple six words were the formula that I proposed they follow and serve as the music for their dance.

In so many ways, those six words were equally as critical in my growth as a parent. Life is about the process, not all the tinsel and tin that we pick up along the way. It's about developing relationships. It's about having meaningful experiences throughout our lives that we can take with us to the grave. Parenting is one of the greatest opportunities bestowed upon us. It provides us not only with opportunities to be nurturers, but with possibilities to find tremendous compassion in our hearts. Anne Lamott, in her book *Operating Instructions: A Journal of My Son's First Year,* states very elegantly that "There really are places in the heart you don't even know exist until you love a child." We believe that it is up to us how we accept and deal with this opportunity.

Introduction to the Parent-Child Dance

Having children and raising a family should be the greatest joy in one's life. However, to bolster something that is that significant requires tremendous responsibility and patience. Parenting is hard work, but the payoff is priceless. Most would say there are no regrets, but also realize that becoming a true family is hard work. As parents, our role must be to provide a strong foundation for our children, so that they can eventually grow up to become self-sufficient adults. However, just like everything in life, all children are different, some requiring more support than others. Parenting is like a fluid, coordinated dance between a parent and child. The metaphor of a dance is used here to represent the interaction between the child and parent. The more seamless the movements are between parent and child, the more graceful the interaction. When a parent takes the lead or decides to share it, over time with practice, the dance can be smooth and effortless.

The parent-child relationship is sometimes like an "interpretive dance," where the choreography is more than just synchronous movements, rich with individual meanings, personal symbolism, and sometimes spontaneous emotion. Dancing well together may not always imply or even require parallel movement. However, it does require an appreciation for individual aesthetic expression, tolerance for nuance and difference, as well as the simple joy of moving together. All of these factors are tied together strongly. They help us respect the unique contributions that each of us brings to the dance.

However, when the child is unintentionally allowed to take the lead, the parent-child dance may appear more rocky and unstable. This often occurs when the parent is unclear and at odds with his/her role. The ensuing battle for the lead may cause disharmony in the relationship and the dance. Parenting is a lifelong commitment to learning how to lead the dance without stepping on your child's toes. It takes patience, thoughtfulness, skill, and commitment. This book is designed to explain the concept of the parent-child dance and act as a catalyst for encouraging all of you to begin your journey in making positive changes in your child's life. The book will also provide a recipe for proactive parenting that will help all parents become more effective in relating to their children. A major emphasis within our writing will focus on explaining and discussing consistent and reliable behavioral solutions that can be put into place. Additionally, throughout the book, attention will also be given to several other meaningful topics including parenting tips for teenagers, strategies for a richer home life and establishing friendships, as well as ideas to build resilience in your sons and daughters.

One of the unique aspects within the various chapters will be our approach to let our readers inside the minds of the parents and children we will be using as examples. Vignettes will not only describe behavioral challenges that parents may be experiencing, they will also incorporate both the parent's and the child's internal dialogue. These insights will be utilized to help all of you appreciate what a child may be thinking (not saying) about their parent's style of responding. Attention will also be given to perhaps what a parent's internal dialogue may be in both successful and frustrating situations. Highlighting the internal dialogue should allow you the opportunity to view the outcome of our teaching strategies, as well as illustrate how parents and children may think throughout the process.

Using the dance metaphor to explain our relationship with our children is clearly a logical choice. It identifies the importance of understanding the underlying interaction between a parent and child and how that interaction either enhances or impedes a child's behavior. We conceive a parent-child interaction akin to a dance because it involves how both parents and children learn to move and respond to one another. Some of us will be more elegant and graceful, while others will be perhaps a little more awkward and inept. Eventually, we will all develop our own style. This book entails learning about your flair. The concepts and suggestions given will provide you with ideas of how to make adjustments to your moves so you can be more in sync with your children. With practice and better understanding, you will become more confident in your parental dance. Let's hope it is a dance style that you feel confident and comfortable with.

Some of us may like ballroom dancing while others may prefer salsa, line, or hip-hop. As with dancing, there are various types of parenting styles. The genre of the dance isn't as relevant as making sure the choice of parenting style works for you. To help expand your awareness and competencies of dance choices, you may need to conduct a bit of research. In your inquiry, you should learn about the range of potential parenting alternatives (dance choices) that are out there. Alternative options of the parent-child dance may be a refreshing option. The same premise holds true with what you will be reading in upcoming chapters. The strategies in upcoming chapters may influence your present style of dance. Who knows what will happen? Once you become more comfortable with your new moves, the sky is the limit.

Parenting, like dancing, must be practiced so we can become more effective with our moves. We need to learn to become more comfortable with our moves and patient with change; these efforts will help boost our confidence. You cannot be expected to dance like Patrick Swayze or Beyonce right away. It takes years of practice to gain such proficiency. Allow yourself to fumble a few times and don't get discouraged; your patience and tenacity will pay off.

Ironically, some parents don't even realize their own behavior (or lack thereof) may be the culprit of negative outcomes. In one situation, a mother of a young high school student was complaining that her daughter constantly argued with her when she gave certain responses to her behaviors. The daughter began to challenge her mother, claiming it wasn't fair when she tried to change her behavior and was still hit with consequences. Typically, the daughter wore down her mom and eventually convinced her to relent. When I talked with the mother, she shared that she was a single child herself and had difficulty following through. "I guess I don't have a backbone to consistently follow through," she said. It isn't surprising that the outcome she often experienced with her daughter was constantly negative. The dance between this mother and daughter was robust and filled with anger. On the other hand, another couple with three children recently talked about how they are now beginning to realize their impact on their children's behavior. They recently shared they noticed that when they were consistent with their boys, and they knew the expectations, they followed the directions given. "It is the consistency and the predictability of what we are requesting that seems to make the difference," they noted. More importantly, you have to remember that you also need to reward and recognize their good behavior when they're just being good, not exceptionally great. This seems to motivate them to cooperate more and feel good about the outcomes.

Both of these examples exemplify the importance of parents' recognizing their contributions to the dance. Lack of being consciously aware of good or bad behavior can have negative repercussions on the interaction. Children need to realize that their parents mean what they say and will act accordingly. They also need to recognize that their parents will make an effort and reward their good behavior and not just focus on what they are doing wrong. When one gives attention to the behaviors that need to change, children begin to realize that they can get what they desire in a cooperative manner. Rearing children with consistency helps them understand predictability and act accordingly.

It is important to appreciate that the more seamless the movements between parent and child, the more graceful the interactions will be. When you are more comfortable in taking the lead or personally decide to share, over time and with practice, the dance can become smooth and effortless. We believe that one of the miscalculations some parents make is when they unintentionally allow the child to take the lead in the parent-child dance. An example of a miscalculation of behavior is when a child misbehaves to get a desired outcome and the parent reluctantly gives in. This may promote the behavior rather than extinguish it. This misstep may cause rocky and unstable interactions. The battle that ensues for the lead may cause disharmony in the relationship and the dance. The dance between a child and a parent may need to be adjusted over the years. An effective parent attends and adjusts to these needs as his/her child moves through adolescence, pre-adulthood, and even into adulthood. The dance may begin as a waltz, but inevitably will take on different forms as parent and child travel through this developmental journey together. For instance, when parenting a preschool-aged child, the process may be highly directive. This style of parenting may be refocused in the teen years as the adolescent searches for more independence.

As stated earlier, bringing up our children is a lifelong commitment to learning how to lead without stepping on our children's toes. It takes our patience and thoughtfulness. It also takes our willingness and commitment to learn various parenting strategies that best meet our child's developmental age and social maturity. This chapter is designed to explain the concept of the parent-child dance and the interactions that take place to foster quality interactions.

The Story of the Bamboo Tree: A Lesson for Parenting

Parenting does take patience and hard work. In fact, sometimes the result of our hard work may not be quickly noticed, but over time and with nurturing, a change will be discerned. The process can be similar to the growth of the Chinese Bamboo Tree. After the seeds of the tree are planted and well taken care of with watering, it will fail to sprout even an inch after the first year. If you didn't know anything about this type of tree, you could become very discouraged about all the efforts with minimal progress. But patience is a real virtue with this plant. It takes approximately five years for you to begin to see growth. Amazingly, during the fifth year the tree shoots up, in some cases beyond 80 feet. We could apply this metaphor of growth to the changes that we sometimes observe in our own children. Over the course of our child's life, just like the growth of a bamboo tree, we may not notice the impact of what we're doing. However, with continued diligence and patience, over time the fruits of our efforts begin to emerge and we recognize the difference.

Denis Waitley notes that the "greatest gift to give children are the roots of responsibility and wings of independence." Ultimately, we have to promote independence in our children. Our children will have to learn to take care of themselves at some point in their lives. It behooves us to help them learn independence developmentally, so the expectations won't surprise them as they age and become adolescents. Our ultimate goal of being parents is to prepare our children to become self-sufficient adults. Our children will become our legacy to the future that will be shaped by our efforts. So here's to the dance. Let the music begin.

Becoming a Parent

Like it or not, becoming a parent is life changing. Our daily routines and existence typically change when children come into play. When we are young and unattached, we are only responsible for ourselves. Adding children to the equation can make things more complicated because we have more people to contend with and people who depend on us. Often, parents prioritize their efforts. Many consider their children's needs beyond their own, but should balance fulfilling their own well-being with that of others. It is not uncommon to hear parents tell others about all of the sacrifices they have had to make in order to support their children. However, in the same breath, most will tell you they have no regrets. The knowledge that their children's life is better seems to make things more worthwhile. In reality, our lives can become busier and more complicated when we become responsible for another. But the blessings (sometimes with heartache and tears) that come in return make it worthwhile. These are priceless opportunities.

No one is promised a bed of thornless roses, and the journey of parenting may be filled with episodes that leave us feeling frustrated, angry, disappointed, and sad. These are the periods that we don't like to think about. But we need to realize that all of us will experience days that our patience will be tested and our hearts will feel like they are breaking. Collectively, all these days, both good and bad, are the moments that we call parenting. They will represent our own personal landscape of opportunities that we will have a hand in cultivating. We must expect that there will be ups and downs similar to any merry-go-round experience. The ride of parenting will either enrich or deplete our souls, most often a combination of both. Hopefully, our experiences will leave us feeling fulfilled with the knowledge that we have left our imprint into the future. George Santayana once elegantly stated that parents "lend to their children their experiences of life as well as a vicarious memory and in return children will endow their parents with a vicarious memory." Our children will allow us the opportunity to help create a life while also enriching our own. Our children will make our lives richer with experiences that are indescribable.

Why Become an Active Parent?

Perhaps one of the major reasons why people become so actively engaged as parents is because of the strength of familial love. There is nothing like sharing and giving love to one's children. As Aubrey recalls, "When my youngest son, Corey, was a very young child, he had a personally heart-warming relationship with a peach-faced lovebird named Coshi. Corey adopted Coshi in 1990, and the bond between the two of them was remarkable. Corey was only in preschool at the time and they became inseparable. It was probably one of the most remarkable relationships that I've ever witnessed with regards to a young boy growing up alongside an animal. As I wrote a few years back in *Afternoons with Puppy* and recently expanded in a new book entitled *Our Faithful Companions,* "Wherever Corey went, the bird tagged along. She would hang on his shirt as they went out to play. I used to get a kick out of watching Corey come to the kitchen in the morning. There he would be marching into breakfast with Coshi dangling on his shirt top. It was a sight to see. We even called some of his shirts 'Coshi's shirts,' because they were slightly chewed around the neck. It was inspiring to see how gentle this rambunctious young preschooler could be with a tiny bird, and how they could play together—something we don't normally associate with a child and a bird."

The family has so many fond memories of the two of them. One of the favorite recollections was how he would drive her around in his small batmobile car. They were a real pair. You had to be there to appreciate the moments watching Corey push this tiny bird in a little toy car. He would gently place her on the seat of the vehicle and slowly push her around the floor. She was so attentive. Sadly, Coshi passed on many years ago, killed by a stray cat. It almost feels like yesterday that Corey mourned her loss, I was sitting right by his side and supporting him. Years later when he graduated from elementary school, he sent his dad a letter letting him know how important it was to him that his dad had taken the time to help him through that difficult episode. Being an active parent is being there for one's children in both good and difficult times.

Long before parents consider the steps they have to take to effectively dance with their child, they typically spend some time considering why they should become a parent. Unfortunately, why one wants to be a parent isn't often discussed. In many ways, it seems to be an expected rite of passage, but some people are more prepared and willing to take on their roles as parents. It is our opinion that parenting is the greatest opportunity for any adult to have. It is the chance to make a difference in another life, but that adult needs to be committed to being engaged. We often hear others say they wished they had done things before that really mattered. Some regret not having spent more time cultivating their relationships with their children. It is hard to imagine that in a blink of an eye, children grow up. Unfortunately, times tarries forward and although we can learn from our past, we cannot regain it.

The song written by Harry Chapin in 1974, *"Cat's in the Cradle,"* resonates this sentiment, and that time lost may never be found. The song is about a child who yearns for his father's attention. Unfortunately, the father has other priorities and always puts off his son and tells him he will play with him later. As they both age, the father begins to want to spend time with his son but now it is the son who is too busy. He turned out to be just like his father. The lesson that is clearly articulated is to be there for your family, and if you're not, they won't be there for you. Hopefully for most of us, we will cherish and recognize the gifts that our children are to us, while we have that chance.

Luther Vandross and Richard Marx, in their song "Dance with My Father," express the importance of parenting as they grieve for one more chance to dance with a father who has died (actually it was Vandross' father who passed away). In one of the stanzas in the song Vandross sings:

If I could get another chance
Another walk, another dance with him
I'd play a song that would never ever end
How I'd love, love, love to dance with my father again

The truth is, as parents we will always be with our children. Our imprint may be a blessing for the child or may have adverse effects. Sure all of us will have rough spots, but if we have a positive impact helping our children grow up and become responsible adults, we will have done our job and trained future dance instructors.

In so many ways being an active parent is all about giving and perhaps being responsible for the needs of others and at times putting those needs beyond one's own. Being a parent is all about enjoying the time that parents have with their children. They grow up way too fast, and our opportunities to impact their childhoods are time-limited. That is why knowing how to gracefully and effectively dance with one's child is crucial! It will make these precious moments richer and allow us to celebrate the times that we have with our children. We will be able to recognize our important influence that we have had in our family's lives. As the parent-child dance begins, parents are, in fact, the archers that will launch their children's beginnings in life and help set their future directions.

Being in harmony with our family allows us to recognize the possibilities of what we can do to enrich our lives as well as the lives of our youngsters. Our ability to enrich lives is perhaps one of the greatest gifts of being active parents. We all have different reasons for wanting to be a parent. For some, it could be our relationship with our own parents that becomes the impetus of why we want to continue the circle of life. We make it a lifelong goal to be the kind of person they were with us. The nurturing and care that exemplify a strong parent-child relationship cuts both ways. We nurture each other and through that process both parent and child become better people for it.

Types of Parenting: Different Types of Dancing

Parenting, like dancing, comes in different styles. Some of us may be in the mood for salsa dancing while others like line dancing. Dependent on the style of the music that is played, the appropriate dance steps will follow.

We all have our individual styles, but we need to appreciate that we may need to adapt what seems natural in our parenting so that our interactions (dance) with our children will be more fluid and effective.

There are, of course, many variables that could influence our style of parenting beyond how our parents have raised us. We cannot only learn from others, but also profit from our own predisposition to parent based on our personality characteristics. However, how we view parenting and our natural personality may make it difficult to embrace alternative parenting styles. A marine in one parenting class stated that what he was learning in the parenting class was counter to all his training and experience. He was not used to providing motivation for his child through positive attention, praise, and external reinforcement. He had learned to lead others through stern orders and swift punishment for not following orders. Providing reinforcement and positive support was foreign to him. He consciously had to make himself try to be positive. However, once he started a more positive approach to parenting, he was pleasantly surprised at the results. His child became more cooperative and their relationship improved. It is important to recognize your natural predisposition and self-evaluate whether an alternative approach might be a better choice. It is his task. This marine learned a wonderful lesson. His life lesson is reminiscent of the story of Michelangelo's carving of the Florentine Pieta. When asked how he created such beautiful and lifelike figures from a block of marble, Michelangelo responded that the figure lives within the rock and that it was his task to bring it out for all to see.

Bringing up our children is really also about training ourselves. We need to understand how we can contribute positively to get our children to respond favorably. It is a two-way street—a dance so to speak. It is the same way with our children. We are trying to help them become self-sufficient, contributing members of our family.

Before we introduce our suggestions to make these exchanges with your children more consistent and predictable, we are going to briefly showcase various types of parenting styles. Perhaps in reading about them you may see some of these characteristics that you follow in your parenting style. Some of us seem to be more prone to being authoritarian in our style of parenting, while others may find themselves extremely permissive or very democratic. Those who are authoritarian may actually be unrealistically harsh on their children and have unrealistic demands, while those who are permissive may be too lax and don't consistently respond to their child. Those that apply democratic and reliable principles may use the right balance to build healthy relationships.

Typically, parents who are more authoritarian try to control their children. They have a very rigid approach and don't seem as nurturing (Timpano, Keough, Mahaffey, Schmidt, & Abramowitz, 2010). These parents dominate and intimidate their children rather than foster personal growth. For example, how many of you have seen moms or dads in grocery stores or in malls barking orders to their children such as "get over here" or "I'm the parent and know more than you, so you do as I say!"? Although some of the parents believe they get the response that they desire, they do it in a manner that promotes fear and compliance rather than cooperation. In essence, the outcome of this style may produce results that we don't plan for and eventually may lead to resistance.

Amy Chua, in her book *Battle Hymn of the Tiger Mother,* talks about a "Tiger Mom" which amplifies an extremely rigid and strict interaction that restricts a child's social life and demands excellence. Chua believes that being strict and verbally and emotionally abrasive will help children become stronger so they can rise above life's disappointments. Parents whose style follows this premise are driven towards excellence without regard to the emotional scars it may cause. Although we too believe in helping children achieve excellence, we are not as comfortable applying such stringent expectations. We believe that there may be other ways to motivate one's children without distancing them. Nevertheless, it is important to point out that some parenting styles are products of cultural traditions and are very hard to break. What is "acceptable" parenting in some countries or cultures can be significantly different from American values and child-rearing practices.

Another parenting style is the permissive parent who may appear laid back and too lax on rules and expectations. Parents who dance with this type of style may respond inconsistently to their children and lack follow-through. "Jose, I am going to let you stay up late tonight, but I hope tomorrow you will be a better listener to me." This quotation is a perfect example of permissiveness. Relaxing the rules does not teach the child anything and may not get his/her cooperation. In fact, it may produce the complete opposite. The child may be thinking, "I can get her to change her mind, just by acting sweet for a few seconds." Permissive parents often want to be more of a friend to the child than a parent. Sometimes, they can simply be ambivalent and immature, inattentive, preoccupied with work, addicted to substances, etc.

Over the years, both of us have witnessed so many examples of this type of parent. Let's meet Susan, who is a mother of two children: a boy and a girl who are eight and ten respectively. Susan frequently feels frustrated because she asks her children to do their chores but they don't follow through. She's very permissive, and often the children just weasel their way out of doing things. She finds herself constantly asking them over and over again to do what she asks, while at times even losing her temper. In one instance, she asks her children to clear their dishes and put them in the sink. They seem used to this type of request and seem oblivious to her. As they often do, they ignore her request and simply plop down in front of the TV. "We will do it, right after the show Mom," they both announce to Mom. The dishes never get done and eventually, after continual nagging, Susan does the job herself. Permissiveness, although seemingly a friendly approach, often does not incorporate consistency. Without boundaries, children don't acknowledge what parents are expecting them to do. They would prefer to do what they would like.

Some people compare permissive parenting to hovering over their children and, at times, doing most things for them. "Helicopter parents," as Jim Fay (1994) likes to call them, are parents who constantly guide their children through decisions and actions. They make sure the job gets done by micro-managing their children's actions. Although hovering may initially seem helpful, it can make a child feel less competent. Indirectly, we may be sending a child a message that she/he cannot do what we expect. Ironically, hovering over children doesn't only occur when they are young, but also when they grow up to become young adults. It appears that this form of parenting continues throughout the lifetime of the relationship. For example, an article from John Hopkins University identified several basic questions to help parents recognize if they may be helicopter parents to their college student. Here are a few examples from that list:

Are you in constant contact with administrators at your child's school?

Have you ever researched or written a college paper for your child?

Do you frequently intervene if your student has had problems with his roommate?

Do you act as your child's secretary? (i.e., make doctor appointments for him, give him morning wake-up calls, etc.)

Have you ever tried to settle grading disputes for your child more than once?

Have you ever chosen classes for your student to take?

Do you feel bad about yourself if your child makes a mistake?

Unfortunately, beyond the various styles we have already discussed there are parents who just are completely uninvolved in their child's life. Uninvolved parents are those who are simply absent. The scientific evidence seems to identify a host of negative repercussions due to this void, including more of these children getting in trouble with the law, abusing drugs and alcohol, experiencing teen pregnancy, dropping out of school, and having a higher rate of suicide attempts (Mitchell, 2010). Ultimately, lack of involvement has tremendous negative ramifications.

Regardless of the actual parenting orientation, some parents are more consistent in applying their guidelines so that their children know what to expect. Our roles as parents are to help our children navigate through good and bad times. Learning to dance in a more seamless unison will typically help with this challenge. Sometimes the parent must be the dance instructor, while in other instances she/he may take on the role of the dance partner. Finally, in other instances the parent may even act as a disc jockey (i.e., controlling and modifying the interaction within the family).

All Families Are Unique: They All Need Love

What it means to be a family hasn't changed over the years, but what a family looks like today has. Families come in so many variations; some have more resources than others, but in reality, all parents truly have the same job to do. Their role is to bring up their children the best way they can. It is important to realize that we understand this position! All of the materials that will be presented in the upcoming chapters are suitable for all types of parents. The key factors for success are an open mind, a willingness to make a difference, and the energy and tenacity to keep on working (otherwise known as having a great pair of dancing shoes).

Many of you may recall watching the film *Mrs. Doubtfire*. It is a wonderful movie about a family going through a divorce and a father's desperate need to stay in touch with his children. The father eventually dresses up as the nanny so that he can be closer to his children. Robin Williams in the role as a father in the film was remarkable, truly emulating his love for his children in a character that was ever so endearing and entertaining. A favorite moment from the film comes at the end, where his fictitious character, Mrs. Doubtfire, becomes the main star of a TV show. There is also the memorable scene where Mrs. Doubtfire reads a letter to her audience that was received from a child. This is what was written:

Dear Mrs. Doubtfire,

Two months ago my mom and dad decided to separate. Now they live in different houses. My brother Andrew says that we aren't to be a family anymore. Is that true? Did I lose my family? Is there anything that I can do to get my parents back together?

Sincerely,
Katie McCormick

After reading the letter, Mrs. Doubtfire looks deeply into the camera and responds by saying:

Oh my dear Katie.

You know some parents when they're angry, they get along much better when they don't live together, they don't fight all the time, and they can become better people, and much better mommies and daddies for you. And sometimes they get back together and sometimes they don't, dear. And if they don't, don't blame yourself. Just because they don't love each other anymore, doesn't mean they don't love you. There are all sorts of different families, Katie. Some families have one mommy. Some families have one daddy or two families, and some children live with their uncle and aunt, some live in homes in separate neighborhoods, in different areas of the country. And they may not see each other for days or weeks or months, and even years. But if there's love, dear, those are the ties that bind. And you'll have a family in your heart forever."

In so many ways, her sentiment will be reflected throughout our book. We realize that most families are far from perfect, but for many of us, the love and support that we find within our families is what keeps us going. Donna Hedges once said, "Having a place to go—is a home. Having someone to love—is a family. Having both—is a blessing." So as Mrs. Doubtfire wonderfully stated, there are many types of families, and this book is made to discuss the dance for all types of families. The typical American family that one envisioned many years ago is much more complex today. There isn't a typical family per se. Different is the new norm. There are many types of families that we can talk about, but as we noted, at the end of the day it doesn't really matter—we are families. There are blended families, single parent families, same-sex families, families of couples that are cohabitating, families that have children in different homes, and children being brought up by other relatives or friends. The major goal in parenting in all these different types of families is not different. We all want the best for our child! However, being a single parent can be immensely more difficult and challenging. The primary challenge relates to sometimes feeling isolated and always having to be on. When one is a single parent, there isn't another person to pass the buck to! You are the buck.

However, this new generation of children that we are now calling Generation Z seems to be much more individualistic than even the millennial child who preceded them. These children seem to feel more entitled and expect much more from their significant others. They also have very scripted and busy lives and are busy in a variety of organized activities. In a recent article for the *New York Times*, Frank Bruni wrote that he believes that kids these days are sheltered from reality by parents who are "promiscuous" with praise. He believes that these children may "grow up expecting the world to bow at their feet and grant them trophies left and right." (Iverson, 2013). Although this new generation of children could promote some new challenges to the parents of today, the forthcoming strategies we will be discussing are timeless. The ideas that we will share will be easy to integrate in any home, especially if parents are willing to coddle less and teach their children that they are responsible for their own lives!

Who Are Successful Families: A Thought to Consider

Aubrey: Over the years, I have often ended many of my public lectures on parenting with a lovely illusion. Often with my magic I utilize storytelling to shape the impact of the trick and make the experience more meaningful for the audience.

One of my favorite tricks is known as the Beads of Prussia. When I present this, I incorporate the lovely theme song from the film *On Golden Pond* as gentle background music while I spin my tale about our relationship with our children. In my left hand I show the audience an acrylic empty tube and then hold up one of thirteen one-inch wood colored beads (red, green, and yellow). As the music plays, I begin to drop one bead at a time into the tube while explaining how each bead represents a critical element in fostering our bond. Together the collection of beads represents the formula that I believe is needed to establish an optimal bond with our children. In addition to the elements that I traditionally incorporate, I am adding four additional components that were highlighted by the U.S. Department of Health and Human Services in 1989 at a conference they convened to identify qualities of successful families. At the conference, researchers from all over North America were asked to create a list of qualities that they believed promoted successful families. The researchers came up with nine items that were published in a study called "Identifying Successful Families." The original nine qualities were the following: (time together, communication, encouragement, commitment, religion/spiritual well-being, social connectedness, adaptability, appreciativeness and clear rules) Figure 1 incorporates several of the qualities highlighted at the conference but also identifies some of our own thoughts.

So for a few moments, in your own mind, imagine this is the closing of a lecture and you are listening to the opening title music of the film *On Golden Pond* arranged by Dave Grusin. The music captivates you as you listen and you watch this special bond form before you. I begin by explaining that the bond between a parent and a child is very special. However, it only will materialize if we put into it what we expect to get out of it. The recipe hinges on adding all the ingredients. In no specific order, I place the beads into the tube, one after the other.

The first bead represents the importance of attention and time. Attention is the source of sustenance that cultivates our relationships. Attention shouldn't only be given on our own accord. It is a cord that binds us. Our children have their needs and may be in need of attention at times we aren't as willing to share. We need to realize that the greatest gift that you can give your child is time and attention. Healthy time feeds our relationships and helps our children blossom. It is the time that we spend with our children that teaches us to become engaged partners. The more optimal time shared, the more connected we will become.

As I gaze into the audience, I drop the second bead into the tube. The second bead, in essence, represents the care that is needed and required to safeguard our children's well-being. Our relationship requires this sense of responsibility because our children depend on us for their daily needs—not only for today, but for their tomorrows, as well. Our safekeeping is a lifelong commitment that doesn't only cover them when they are young, but also as they mature.

The third bead (which was highlighted in the conference) is our ability to communicate and encourage our children. Successful families communicate frequently and when they interact, they are open and honest. They

Figure 1
Formula for Successful Parenting

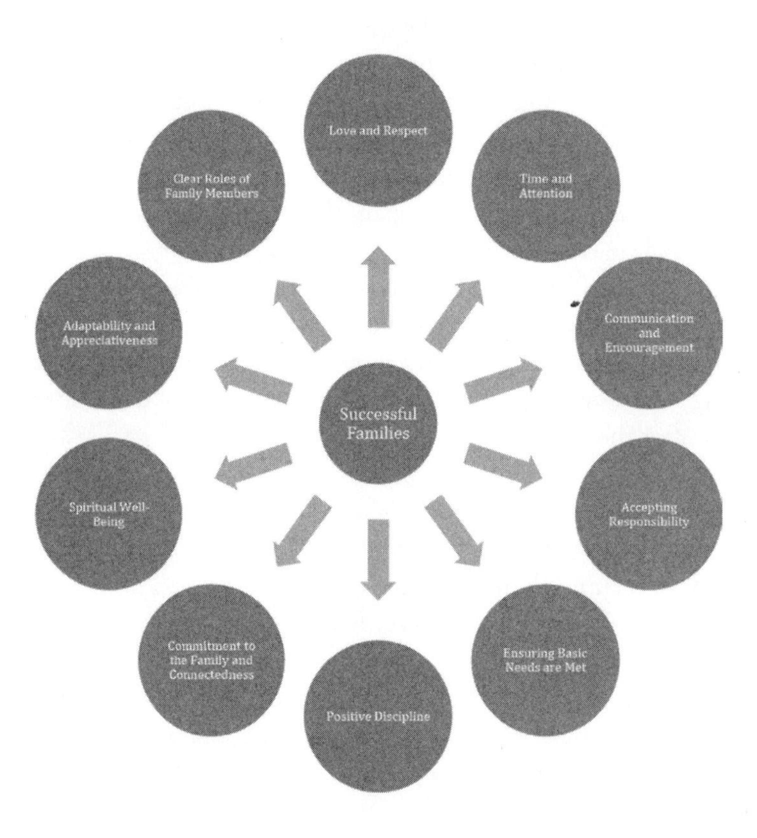

also are encouraging to one another. They facilitate a manner that allows every member to feel a strong sense of belonging to the family. An encouraging family helps the members develop their talents and strengths.

The fourth element is one that most of us cherish. It is playing and having fun with our children. Having fun can happen at all ages. That is why we have children and, in some ways, is a cornerstone of our relationships. As the old saying notes, "The family that plays together stays together." We all benefit from this interaction.

I traditionally pause at this point and then drop in the next three beads simultaneously. The fifth bead represents the importance of taking care of our children's basic needs (their health, shelter, and sustenance). These are, in reality, critical elements of daily living. They aren't flamboyant, but yet they are necessities for life.

The eighth bead dropped into the tube captures our commitment to the family and recognizes our need to be connected to others. (Both of these two ingredients are from the 1989 conference.) Members of families must be committed to each other but also must not be isolated from people outside of the family. Successful families need a strong social network outside their homes.

The ninth bead relates to understanding our roles in the family. Defining our roles and their significance is critical to family dynamics and cohesiveness.

The next two elements combine to form the tenth bead and relate to spiritual well-being and the ability to adapt and conform. Spiritual well-being promotes compassion and love for others, and helps us strive to find the greater good in all of us. The second element represents an important ingredient in all of our families in its ability to adapt and handle times of stress and difficulty.

Discipline and teaching, the eleventh bead, is crucial for an effective relationship. It is perhaps one of the most important elements in our formula of building our very special bond. Many people misunderstand the term "discipline" as being cruel or harsh. In essence, the true meaning of discipline is training through eyes of a disciple. We have to learn to co-exist. We need to teach our children to co-exist. That is one of our major messages in this book. The dance includes ways that we incorporate the steps that will teach our children to move more effectively.

This leads us to the last bead. The final ingredient in our strand could have been dropped in the first, but I always choose it for the last. It is the most potent ingredient that ties the bond together. It is the simplest of all. It's love and respect. It's devotion. It's our willingness to engage and share our hearts with another special being that makes this bond complete. It is also the element that ties us together.

At this point, the theme song is about to end and just then, I say that it is our mutual love and respect that ties us together, I toss the beads into the air. Astonishingly, and to the surprise of the audience, they are magically strung together to form a necklace. The strand of beads helps the audience crystallize how all these ingredients blend together. The visual effect usually gets them to clearly see my message. It is a message that promotes the idea that a healthy combination of all of these elements makes the bond between parent and child unbreakable!

Final Thoughts

No one ever said parenting would be easy, but so many of us have learned to appreciate how priceless the experience can be. It is the totality of these experiences that we are focusing upon, and our intentions are to simplify how parents can get the most out of this opportunity. We want to make your dance with your child seamless. We also want you to understand the steps that you need to take to become more a competent and relaxed parent. Most importantly, we want you to enjoy this journey while you have the opportunity.

It takes one step to begin your new journey towards parenting and we believe we have the map to get you there, so let the music and dancing begin. Let's paraphrase what Richard Paul Evans once stated, Dance. Dance for the joy and breath of childhood…Embrace the moment before it escapes from your grasp… And in the end, we must ask ourselves what we have given our children… And was it enough? This is a question we must constantly ask while challenging ourselves to strive for improvement.

References

Chua, A. (2011) *Battle Hymn of the Tiger Mom*. New York: Penguin Press.

Fine, A. & Eisen, C. (2007) *Afternoons with Puppy*. West Lafayette, IN: Purdue University Press.

Fine, A. (2014). *Our Faithful Companions: Exploring the Essence of Our Kinship with Animals*. Crawford, CO: Alpine Publications Inc.

Iverson, K. (2013, November 25). Millennials No Longer Laziest, Worst Generation. *Brooklyn Magazine*. Retrieved from http://www.bkmag.com/2013/11/25/millennials-no-longer-laziest-worst-generation/

John Hopkins University. (n.d.). *Are You a Helicopter Parent?* Retrieved from http://web.jhu.edu/reslife/parents/Are%20You%20a%20Helicopter%20Parent.pdf

Lamott, A. (1993). *Operating Instructions: A Journal of My Son's First Year*. New York: Ballantine.

Mitchell, P. (2010). Helicopter parents: Is there ever too much parenting? *Children's Voice, 19(6)*, 33.

Timpano, K., Keough, M., Mahaffey, B., Schmidt, N., & Abramowitz, J. (2010). Parenting and obsessive-compulsive symptoms: Implications of authoritarian parenting. *Journal of Cognitive Psychotherapy, 24(3)*, 151–164.

Waitley, D. (n.d.). *The greatest gifts you can give your children are the roots of responsibility and the wings of independence*. In BrainyQuote's online quotation database. Retrieved from http://www.brainyquote.com/quotes/quotes/d/deniswaitl165021.html

SECTION II

Introduction to Section II

In this section we will describe a wide range of proven effective approaches to motivate your child to comply with your requests and to do his/her best. Sprinkled within all of these chapters will be a unique dimension that we believe will enhance our presentation of the materials. We will often capture children's and parents' internal thinking so that you as a reader will be able to appreciate first-hand insights on how people think about behavioral change. We will provide you with insights into how children may think about our efforts in trying new parenting strategies as well as typical thoughts that parents may have as they respond to their child's behavior.

In our thirty-plus years of meeting with parents, we have become extremely conscious of how parents may respond to the strategies we suggest and are aware of how this may impact how they apply these alternatives. By hearing some of these typical thoughts (that parents and children may share), it may help you have a deeper understanding of how best to apply the material we will share with you.

We conceptualize parenting as a dance because it involves both the parents' and the child's reciprocal reactions to each other. As clinicians, we have heard the many thoughts and reactions that children have expressed when their parents suddenly change their parenting style. Hearing these thoughts by capturing the viewpoint of the child can help you more clearly understand and accept how children typically adjust to the changes parents make in their styles of parenting.

In this section (chapters 2–6) we will introduce strategies for clearly communicating, teaching, and prompting your child's behavior. Our descriptions will include a wide range of approaches that we have found extremely powerful and effective with most children. Additionally, we will also discuss strategies that are designed to decrease dangerous, oppositional, and socially inappropriate behavior. To help with applying these ideas, we have developed several forms for application. These forms are incorporated to help you plan how you can implement each strategy and to plan ahead.

Finally, as parents, you will also be able to learn how to avoid missteps in implementing the parenting strategies highlighted. Each of these strategies will be introduced through a brief scenario that will be presented. A solution applying one of the strategies previously noted will be explained after hearing the parent and child's viewpoint (as we alluded to earlier) to get a clear understanding of their internal thinking. The process of illustrating their points of view will also be utilized to highlight the difference in their thinking after the strategies have been applied.

Finally, Chapter 6 will introduce specific strategies to help children with friendships. The materials will expose you to numerous methods of how to help your child get along with others. The ideas are based on our experience in working with children as well as helping their parents apply the strategies to support this process.

Disclaimer:

The strategies presented in this section take time to work. It may take several weeks to a month of consistently implementing the strategies in each section to see a significant change. One of the greatest missteps is expecting immediate change and giving up too soon. If you have patience and persistence you will successfully help your child make needed changes in his/her behavior.

CHAPTER 2

Learning Basic Steps: Understanding Techniques That Make Leading Easier

Over the course of the last three decades, both of us have intimately worked with families, helping them develop their parenting skills. We specialize in understanding methods of how to encourage positive interactions between parents' and their children. Throughout the following chapters, we will provide parents with suggestions on how they can foster more harmonious households and be in step with their children. We will utilize our years of experience to provide parents with effective guidelines and strategies to foster cooperation and decrease conflict in the home. The end result is that parents will become more confident and effective.

The metaphor of the Parent-Child Dance is designed to remind parents that parenting is a reciprocal relationship. Parents are attempting to influence their child's behavior, and their child's response is affecting their parents behavior. It is important to realize that parenting should not only be about what parents want their child to do, but must take into consideration what the child wants. Parents must try to consider their child's perspective if they are going to be successful in parenting. Resistance to change is normal and should not be viewed as unnatural. It is also important that parents consider what their child needs to do in order to be able to be successful, and not just what the parents want them to do.

To enhance your understanding of the parenting strategies presented in the upcoming chapters (2–6) we will also present insights from a parent and child's perspective. We have taken creative license in writing the child's point of view from the perspective of an adult reflecting on their childhood experiences. Having a clear understanding of both the view of the parent and the child will enhance your understanding of what to expect when trying new approaches to parenting.

All of the parenting strategies presented in this chapter will focus on how to set your child up for success. This chapter will provide the impetus for building a strong parenting foundation. We believe that attention must first be given to the components of good teaching since parents are teachers and need to understand basic teaching strategies. You will gain insight into the importance of breaking a task down into smaller manageable steps and teaching these sequentially. You will also learn how modeling behavior can be an effective and efficient way of teaching new behaviors. You will next learn the value of providing visual prompts to help your child remember what he/she has learned. You will also gain insight into the importance of giving clear effective commands to ensure that your child understands what he/she is being asked to do. Finally, you will learn that giving your child at least five seconds to respond to a direction and allowing them ten minutes to stop a favorite activity may increase the likelihood that your child will comply with you. For organization, the chapter will be divided into the following short sections, allowing for clarity and building on each ingredient:

A. Teaching Is Not a Magic Trick
B. Words Are Only as Good as the Visual Images That Accompany Them
C. Signs in the Right Direction
D. Say What You Mean and Mean What You Say
E. Posting and Simplifying Rules
F. The Five-Second Rule and the Ten-Minute Countdown

A. Teaching Is Not a Magic Trick

Parents often fail to recognize how difficult it is for a child to learn new skills. They may have unrealistic expectations for their child. This section will give insight into the importance of breaking tasks down into manageable steps and teaching your child each step until they master it, before moving on to the next step.

Scenario 1: Sam and Carla are having difficulty teaching their son how to tie his shoes. They have tried unsuccessfully for weeks to teach him this skill. Before we present a solution to the situation, let's hear first-hand what the parents and child are experiencing.

Parent Viewpoint

We have tried for weeks to teach Carlos to tie his shoes. Often he just cries and complains that he cannot do it. We have tried everything! We have slowly gone through the steps of how a shoe is tied and even modeled those steps for him. We have tried talking him through the process of tying his shoes, but he just doesn't seem to get it. We know that this is just one of the many things we will need to teach him and we want to learn how best to do it.

Child Viewpoint

Now I know my parents don't have a teaching credential, but telling me one time and showing me once how to tie my shoes does not constitute teaching. I am sure my dad and mom did not learn to drive that way. Well, it doesn't work! To me it was like a magic show where my parents said a bunch of words and did a sleight of hand trick and the shoes were tied. After this display of what I thought was magic they said, "Now you try it." I panicked! They acted like it was easy and now I was supposed to perform the same magic. With much coaxing, I gave it a try. I twisted the laces every which way and threw my hands up like a good magician and hoped for the best. Nothing happened, my shoelaces just flopped to the side. My parents looked at me with disappointment. I immediately felt dumb. I could tell that they felt that any child my age should be able to tie a shoe using the tried and true method of one-trial-learning. I am ashamed of myself and I feel like crying. My parents got me Velcro shoes.

Solution 1: Teaching Is Not a Magic Trick – Break the Steps Down

Parents are their child's first and most important teachers. Teaching is a skill that often does not come naturally. Part of being an effective parent is being an effective teacher. Teaching requires love and affection, nurturing, patience, keen observation, and the ability to analyze a task and break it down into smaller, teachable steps. What does your child need to do to sequentially complete the task? What skills does he/she have and what skills does he/she need to learn? It is rare that your child will have absolutely no skills to complete the task. We need to build on the skills he/she already has and train him/her in the skills that are missing or weak.

The final step is motivating your child to be eager to learn what you are trying to teach. Learning new tasks can be difficult and challenging. Whenever something is difficult, the natural tendency is to avoid it. Children need motivation to make the effort necessary to learn and practice a new task. They need to practice the task until it is mastered. When something is difficult, children will experience stress and prefer to avoid the task completely. Why would you do something that highlights your weaknesses? It makes sense that we need strong motivation to practice the skill until we master it and no longer feel incompetent. After each trial the child should be given genuine praise and positive reinforcement for his/her efforts.

It is also extremely important that the parent as teacher remain calm and supportive. Remember, while the task may be easy for you, it is difficult and challenging for your child. The art of motivating your child will be covered in the next chapter.

Sam and Carla have been trying to teach their child, Carlos, to tie his shoes with little success. They know that he is old enough to tie his shoes and that most kids his age have already learned to tie their shoes. Unfortunately, they have given up and bought Velcro shoes. Sam and Carla have now learned a new approach to teaching and are ready to try again. Let's hear from Sam, Carla, and Carlos now that the parents have learned and are ready to apply the steps for teaching new skills.

Parent Viewpoint

We recently learned that our approach might not be the best. Teaching is a skill and we need to work at it. We had unrealistic expectations. Shoe tying requires many smaller steps and showing him the whole process seems to be overwhelming. We broke the task down into smaller individual steps and then strung them together as he learned each step. We praised Carlos and rewarded him for attempting each new step. Breaking the steps down allowed him to have small successes as he learned each new step. This seems to work! Carlos seems more relaxed. He smiles and is more willing to learn.

Child Viewpoint

Wow, this new way seems to work! I actually can do this. Breaking up the steps is much easier. We practiced each small step a bunch of times until I could do it perfectly. I really felt good when they praised me. They then taught me each new step one at a time and we practiced until I could finally tie my shoe by myself.

B. Words Are Only as Good as the Visual Images That Accompany Them

Modeling is a powerful way in which children learn new behavior. Children learn more from what we do than what we say. If what we say does not match what we do, they are more likely to do as we do.

Scenario 2: David and Beth are concerned that their son Alan is rude and aggressive when talking with them and others. They are not sure why this is happening. They have not looked at their own behavior as a possible reason for Alan's behavior. Let's listen.

Parent Viewpoint

Lately the only time we feel comfortable with our child is when he is sleeping. That is a sad thing to say, but true. He yells and demands things from us until he gets what he wants. He will grab things out of our hands rather than ask us politely for them. He pushes past us to go outside even when we tell him he can't leave the house. He has even resorted to hitting us if he doesn't get his way. It seems that we are raising a monster.

Child Viewpoint

What they say to me does not always match what I see them do. For example, sometimes I get mad at another kid for taking my toys from me. I automatically hit him. My parents get angry when I hurt someone and yell, "We don't hit other people!" as they spank me. I understand what they are saying, but the mental image says it all. We do hit when we are mad. I seem to be learning a lot of bad habits. If you think about it, it's kind of funny. My parents don't listen to their own advice: "Don't raise your voice to me!" (As they are yelling), "Watch your mouth!" (As they are swearing), "Clean up after yourself!" (As they toss their clothes everywhere). I am constantly getting in trouble for being the spitting image of my parents. "Do as I say not as I do" is wishful thinking when it comes to kids. It would certainly be easier for me if they showed me what to do rather than using all those words to tell me what to do.

Solution 2: Words Are Only as Good as the Visual Images That Accompany Them

One of the most powerful and efficient ways in which children learn new behavior is through modeling. Children watch everything we do and try to imitate what they see. Imagine how many things your child learns by simply imitating what they see. If they can learn a complex task through observation we do not need to go through the time-consuming process of breaking each task down and teaching each component.

Children learn most of what they know through modeling. This is a double-edged sword. They also imitate behavior we do not want them to learn. The very behavior that we may want to change may have been learned through imitating our behavior.

David and Beth are very upset with their child's aggressive, rude behavior. They have tried everything in their repertoire to stop their child's behavior, and nothing has worked. They are desperate and finally decide to look for an alternative way of changing Alan's behavior by modeling the behavior for him. They love their child but find it hard to be around him when he is rude and even aggressive with them. Let's hear what happens when David and Beth begin to model the behavior they want to see in Alan.

Parent Viewpoint

We need to control our actions if we expect Alan to do the same. The more he became rude, the more we yelled at him and spanked him. Our behavior seemed to escalate with his behavior. Once we became aware that being role models wasn't just an abstract goal but actually affected our child's behavior, we took a good long look at ourselves. We had to admit that we were often rude to one another and frequently raised our voices to make sure we made our point. We were not much different from our child. We made a pact to stop all aggressive, rude behavior and start modeling what we wanted Alan to do. Wow, what a difference! Within a week we began to see a change. Not completely, but there was a glimmer of hope.

It has been two months since we started our effort to change our rude aggressive behavior. We now model more civil responses and our child is no longer rude and aggressive. Sure, on occasion he raises his voice or tends towards aggressive behavior, but that is not any different from other children his age. He is much happier and we are ecstatic. This has helped not only our relationship with our child, but with one another.

Child Viewpoint

Recently, my parents have begun to change what they do. They no longer raise their voices and have stopped spanking me. I feel calmer and don't feel angry all the time. I notice that I am also starting to ask for things in a nice way. This works for me. We are getting along better and spending more time together. I like what I see and want to be more like them.

C. Signs in the Right Direction

When you give your child a direction or ask your child to complete a complex sequence of tasks, what you ask him/her to do vanishes. He/she can easily forget what you asked him/her. A visual reminder, such as a chart, poster, or pictures, is a permanent reminder of the sequence of tasks you asked him/her to do. These visual reminders can be referred to over and over again, making the visual illustration more effective than the spoken request.

Scenario 3: Chris and Clara are stymied as to how to get Michelle to remember her morning routine. They know she is bright, but she just can't seem to learn a morning routine. Let's listen to Chris, Clara, and Michelle describe the situation.

Parent Viewpoint

We are extremely frustrated with Michelle. She is a very sweet girl who tries to please us. Each morning we have to tell her what to do. We let her know what she is supposed to do before she goes to school. Invariably she forgets half of what we told her. It is the same routine each day, but she just doesn't seem to get it. This is so frustrating. We know that we don't handle this very well. We end up yelling at her and she ends up crying and says she's sorry. I don't think she is deliberately trying to defy us, but it sure appears that way.

Child Viewpoint

It's hard to remember all the things my parents want me to do. Once they say them, the words disappear into thin air. They are just gone. If my parents use a lot of words it is really hard to remember. My parents sometimes yell at me for forgetting. They take me by the hand and stand over me while I complete the task I forgot. Sometimes I feel sad because they are disappointed in me and this makes me cry.

Solution 3: Signs in the Right Direction

Parents establish routines that they expect their child to follow. They explain what they want in varying degrees of specificity and expect their child to remember. One way to help your child achieve success in following a routine is to give him/her a visual chart that shows step-by-step what you want him/her to do. He/she can draw pictures depicting each step, or you can actually take pictures of your child completing the sequence. It is important to include your child in creating the chart to help get his/her buy-in.

At first, walk him/her through each step to make sure he/she understands what is expected of him/her. Have him/her tell you what he/she is supposed to do. Don't assume that because he/she looked at the picture that he/she understands. Next, refer him/her to the chart and reinforce him/her for completing each task independently. Referring to the chart will reduce the need for you to constantly nag him/her.

Chris and Clara came to us for advice on how to get their daughter, Michelle, to follow a routine without having to be told multiple times what to do. Their daughter is extremely bright and they've been frustrated with the fact that she seems to forget what she is supposed to do even though the routine is the same each day. They don't know whether she is being oppositional or really forgets. Let's hear from Chris, Clara, and Michelle about what happens when Michelle is given a chart (see Figure 1) to help her remember her morning routine.

Important note: The chart needs to be made child friendly. Children will be more likely to show interest in the chart if they are involved in creating it. Three strategies that can increase children's interest in the chart are:

1. Have your child draw a picture of them-selves completing each task for use in the chart.
2. Take pictures of them completing each task for use in the chart.
3. Have them decorate the chart.

Figure 1
Morning Routine

	Wake Up
	Brush Your Teeth, Wash Your Face
	Get Dressed
	Eat Your Breakfast

Parent Viewpoint

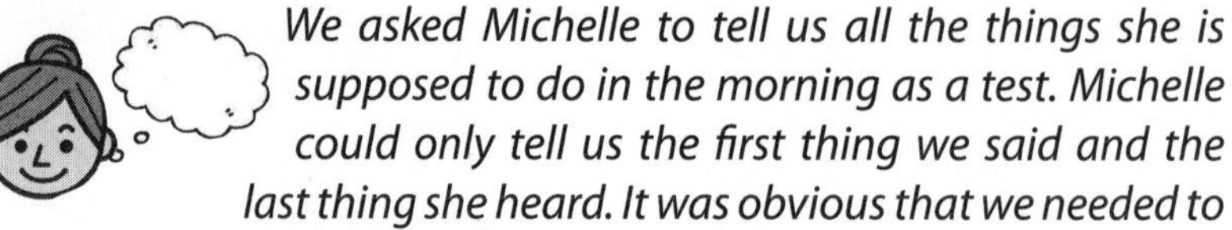

We asked Michelle to tell us all the things she is supposed to do in the morning as a test. Michelle could only tell us the first thing we said and the last thing she heard. It was obvious that we needed to find a way to help her remember what she needed to do. We created a chart and took pictures of her doing each task in sequence and put it on the chart. This made it easier for her to remember what she needed to do. We encouraged Michelle to decorate the chart anyway she wanted. When we involved her in decorating the chart she became more at ease and had buy-in to the chart.

This really worked! Having a chart with pictures to remind her of what she needs to do makes it easier for her. Each time she completes a task we praise her. Now we just have to point to the chart and ask her to check it in the morning to remember what she needs to do instead of nagging her.

It is unbelievable! We can't believe how this simple strategy made it easier for her. Michelle is now independently completing all her tasks. We have stopped nagging her. We can add tasks to her chart if we need her to remember something new we have asked her to do. I guess we were being unrealistic in expecting her to remember all the things we asked her to do on her own.

Child Viewpoint

Sometimes I choose not to do what my parents want me to do because I don't want to stop what I am doing. But sometimes I just forget. The chart is a good reminder that helps me to remember. Having the chart in a place where I can't miss seeing it really helps. It makes me feel good when I remember to do things on my own.

D. Say What You Mean and Mean What You Say

The English language is very complex. Communicating accurately can be a real challenge. Often a child may appear non-compliant when the problem really stems from poor communication. Parents should make sure they say what they mean and mean what they say.

Scenario 4: Michael and Sharon shared with us their frustration with Billy. Billy frequently fails to follow their directions. They are beginning to think that he may need help from a Speech and Language Therapist because he seems to have trouble understanding what they want him to do. They are also confused as to whether he is oppositional or he just doesn't understand what they are asking him. Often, when they ask him to do something he looks confused. Let's hear from Michael, Sharon, and Billy.

Parent Viewpoint

We have been in a constant battle with Billy because he rarely complies with a direction the first time we ask. He looks at us as if we are speaking a foreign language. Even when he does try to follow our directions he only partially completes the task we ask him to do. We know Billy is smart but he may have a problem processing language.

Child Viewpoint

I can't seem to do anything right. I try to do what my parents ask me to do. They get mad at me all the time. My mom says things like, "Let's go clean up your room." I go to my room and wait for her. Twenty minutes later she comes into the room, looks at the condition of the room and chews me out for not cleaning my room. How fair is that? She said, "Let's clean your room." Well, I waited and she took twenty minutes to join me. I guess "let's" means "you." Dad would say, "Wouldn't you like to start your homework now?" Of course I would answer honestly and say "No." He then chews me out for being rude. "How dare I refuse to do my homework?" My parents sometimes say things like, "Why don't you go take care of your room?" I go look at my room and figure I took care of my room. They go into my room several hours later and list all the things I forgot to do in "taking care of my room." I guess they thought I was a mind reader. They tell me ten things to do without taking a breath. I always remember the first and the last thing they said and have no idea what the middle things were.

Solution 4: Say What You Mean and Mean What You Say

In our everyday communications, we often think that we are exceedingly clear in what we are saying. The English language is complex and can be confusing. If the person receiving our communication is unclear as to what we mean, this is an invitation for conflict. Children are often extremely literal and think that we mean exactly what we say. If we are not careful, we can set them up to appear non-compliant. One effective way of prompting children to listen is to start with the phrase "You have a direction to..."

This prompts us to state what we clearly want them to do. Here in Table 1 are a few ineffective directions, how children perceive them and what we actually mean:

Table 1

INEFFECTIVE COMMANDS

"LET'S" COMMANDS

Direction:
Let's clean your room.

Child's interpretation:
We are going to clean the room together.

What we meant:
Clean your room.

QUESTION COMMANDS

Direction:
Wouldn't you like to do your homework?

Child's interpretation:
I have a choice of whether I want to do my homework. No, I don't think I want to do homework.

What we meant:
Do your homework.

LONG CHAIN OF COMMANDS

Direction:
Clean your room, wash your hands, and get ready for dinner, feed the dog, help your mother set the table, and don't forget to put away your skateboard.

Child's interpretation:
Clean your room…

What we meant:
Too many things to remember even for the parent who said them.

VAGUE COMMANDS

Direction:
Take care of your room…

Child's interpretation:
Go into my room and check it out.

What we meant:
Put the clothes on the floor in their appropriate drawer. Make your bed and put your toys in the toy bin.

Giving clear directions increases your child's ability to comply with you.

Parents often get angry because they think that their children are purposely not doing what they were told to do. A simple way to test whether they are ignoring us is to ask them to repeat the directions. If they can't repeat the directions then they weren't listening, didn't understand, or our intended meaning was not clearly expressed by us.

Sharon and Michael have learned through our advice that the problem may be in the words they are using to communicate with Billy. They may not be clear in their directions and are confusing him by how they ask him to do things. They are going to try to change how they phrase their requests so that what they want Billy to do is crystal clear. Let's hear what Sharon, Michael, and Billy think once communication is clear and concise.

Parent Viewpoint

We thought the problem was Billy. Apparently, we need speech and language therapy. We are unclear in our directions and Billy is merely doing what we are literally asking him to do. Our directions are unclear and non-specific. We learned a simple trick. If we give direction to do something, we should start the direction with the phrase, "You have a direction to..." By stating that he has a direction to... we are forced to say what we want him to do. Also, we have to be careful not to string together multiple requests in one long sentence. He may not be able to remember everything we said. We also have a habit of saying "let's" do something when we mean for him to do it. That sounds as if we are going to help him. We really mean for him to do it without our help. We can see where that would be confusing. We also ask him if he would like to do something when it really isn't a choice. The ultimate test of whether he is defying us or just didn't understand us is to ask him to repeat what we said. Of course, we also have to make sure that we haven't fallen into one of the traps of miscommunication. If he can't repeat what we say then he didn't understand the direction.

Once we started making sure our directions were easy to understand and were clear in what we expected Billy to do, we were surprised to see that Billy suddenly became more compliant.

Child Viewpoint

I knew something had happened because my parents were suddenly saying what they meant and meaning what they said. "Let's go clean up your room", was now, "You have a direction to clean up your room." Dad stopped asking me if I wanted to do my homework and said, "You have a direction to do your homework now," "Take care of your room" was now, "You have a direction to pick up the clothes off the floor and put them in your dresser." I no longer was being required to be a mind reader. My parents gave me no more than two tasks at a time to remember and complete. This worked well because I could typically remember two assigned tasks from a long list, the first and the last. They also made things much easier for me, and them, by asking me to repeat what I understood about what they had asked me to do. If I couldn't repeat what they said, they simply repeated the direction. Now that I can remember what to do, I feel like a genius.

E. Posting and Simplifying Rules

Parents have rules they expect their child to follow whether they are stated or not. A set of simple clearly written rules posted where the child cannot miss them increases the likelihood that they will follow those rules. In this section, parents will learn how to write reasonable rules that children can follow.

Scenario 5: Kathy and Rick expected Steve to follow their house rules. They were sure he knew what the rules were. They felt that Steve ignored them and deliberately defied them. Let's hear what Kathy, Rick, and Steve have to say.

Parent Viewpoint

We really don't want to write out our house rules for Steve. He already knows them. Steve just chooses not to follow our rules. Things are not going well and we know that we need to try something different beyond nagging and getting angry.

Child Viewpoint

My parents expect me to be able to read their minds. They keep telling me that I am breaking rules when I don't do what they expect me to do. I never know when they are going to get angry with me and accuse me of not following the rules. I frankly don't know what rules they are talking about. I don't like getting into trouble for not following the rules, but how can I follow the rules if I don't know what they are? Somehow they think I should just know what they expect of me. I wish I knew what the rules were so I could follow them and they would stop yelling at me.

Solution 5: Posting and Simplifying Rules

Every household has house rules whether they are implied or stated. Posting home rules can be a very effective way of helping children know what is expected from them. When creating house rules, parents should follow some basic steps. Table 2 lists the basic steps.

Table 2

Posting and Simplifying Rules

1. First, decide on no more than four important rules. You may have many expectations for your child but they are not equally important. The important rules are those rules that create harmony between the parent and child. You want to keep the rules down to no more than four so that they are easy to remember for both you and your child. They should also be rules that are not too difficult for him/her to remember or put into practice. Expectations need to be realistic for the child to implement.
2. State the rules in precise behavioral terms. Always state what you want your child to do. What would you see your child doing if they were following your rule?
3. In the written rule, state what will happen if your child follows the rule and what will happen if they do not follow the rule.
4. Go over the rules with your child and make sure that your child understands the rules and consequences for following or not following the rules.
5. Post the rules in a prominent place where you and your child cannot miss seeing them. Most people choose the refrigerator because each time you get food you can't help seeing the rules.
6. Review the rules for the first week and refer to them often.

Kathy and Rick expected their son Steve to follow their rules. When we asked them what rules they had established for Steve to follow they had to think about it. They stated several vague rules that they said he knew very well but chose to ignore. We asked them what they did when Steve didn't follow their rules and they had trouble explaining specific consequences for not following the rules. They also were not able to tell us what happened when he followed their rules. They said that they really did not feel that they needed to reward him for doing what he was supposed to do. It was clear that they needed to create clear and concise written rules, with praise and rewards for following the rules, and specific clearly stated consequences for failing to follow the rules.

After reviewing the steps in establishing home rules with Kathy and Rick, they decided to try establishing clear written rules with consequences to see if this would improve Steve's behavior. Let's hear what happens when Kathy and Rick write clear and concise rules for Steve to follow.

Parent Viewpoint

We finally had to admit that it made sense that writing the rules down and posting them where we could all refer to them might help. We took the time to write out the rules of the house. There were four rules:

1. *Pick up after yourself*
2. *Speak in a respectful manner*
3. *Finish your meal before watching TV*
4. *Tell us where you are going before leaving the house*

We went over the rules with Steve and gave him a copy. For the first several weeks nothing changed. We began to think that this wasn't going to work. Then it occurred to us that we had forgotten two very important steps, writing consequences and posting the rules where they couldn't be missed. We started paying attention when Steve followed a rule and began praising him. We also made the amount of nightly computer time he could have contingent on the rules he followed. He could earn a maximum of 60 minutes of computer time each night. He could earn 15 minutes of computer time for each rule that he followed. The more rules he followed the more computer time he earned. This seemed to get his attention. After losing several days of computer time he suddenly started following our rules. We no longer have to remind him.

Child Viewpoint

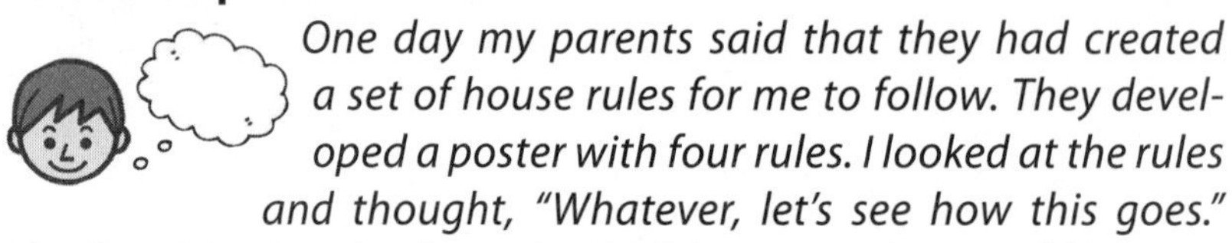

One day my parents said that they had created a set of house rules for me to follow. They developed a poster with four rules. I looked at the rules and thought, "Whatever, let's see how this goes." The first thing I noticed was that it did not say what would happen if I did not follow the rules. It also did not give me a reason to want to follow the rules. As I looked at the four rules I thought, "They're not going to remember these rules and neither am I." I breathed a sigh of relief when they gave me a copy of the rules and put the rules on the counter where no one could see them. If they were serious, they would have posted them on the fridge. Sure enough, they seldom, if ever, referred to the rules and only threatened me if I broke a rule.

I was not following their home rules until suddenly things changed. They stepped it up a notch. They added a reward for following the rules and punishment for not following the rules. My computer time each night depended on the number of rules I followed. Now I knew they were serious because they posted it on the fridge.

F. The Five-Second-Rule and the Ten-Minute Countdown

Parents often expect children to instantly respond to a command. Children are often punished if they do not respond immediately. Within this section, we will discuss the value of the five-second rule. We believe that waiting five seconds after giving a direction before reacting can result in more compliance and avoids unnecessary punishment for non-compliance.

A second problem arises when children are playing a favorite game or activity. Children often throw a tantrum when asked to stop a favorite activity. They need time to wind down. Parents will learn that giving children a ten-minute warning with periodic prompts can prevent children from overreacting when asked to stop doing something they enjoy doing. We compare this warning to a traffic light where yellow means be ready to stop.

Scenario 6: Fred and Juanita find themselves frequently punishing Vince for not following their directions immediately. He also refuses to stop playing with his toys and put them away when they ask him to stop. This

has been escalating and it is affecting their relationship. Fred, Juanita, and Vince share their thoughts with us.

Parent Viewpoint

Vince seems determined to defy us. At least that is how it seems. We ask him to do something and he doesn't do it right away. He also has a bad temper and gets angry with us when he is playing and we ask him to stop playing and follow our directions. We are his parents and he should listen to us when we ask him to do something. We don't like getting mad at Vince but he is constantly challenging us. We love Vince but it is getting really hard to be around him when he doesn't listen to us. We're sure it isn't pleasant for him either.

Child Viewpoint

My parents have added an expectation of me when they give me directions, "instantaneous compliance, in a flash, now, from my lips to your fast twitch muscles." They must think I am Superman and can move faster than a speeding bullet. Well guess what? This new expectation has resulted in many battles. What a setup!

Solution 6: The Five-Second Rule and the Ten-Minute Countdown

Parents often have unrealistic expectations. They not only take it for granted that their child will comply with their expectations, but want that compliance to happen instantaneously. They give a direction and get angry when their child does not comply immediately. This results in multiple punishments, yelling, and sometimes spanking. The five-second rule may improve the situation. If parents wait five seconds after giving their child a direction he/she is more likely to comply with their request. Beyond five seconds he/she is not as likely to comply.

Although it is realistic to give a child five seconds to respond to a direction, we need to recognize that this may be difficult if he/she is in the middle of a game or activity. Abruptly asking a child to stop a favorite activity is difficult and unfair to him/her. It often leads to tantrums and aggressive behavior. He/she needs advance warning so he/she will have time to wind down and stop what he/she is doing. We believe that letting him/her know (like a yellow traffic light) that he/she is expected to stop in ten minutes helps him/her be able to stop. Remind him/her periodically that the ten minutes are almost up. It is important to assure him/her that he/she can go back to what he/she was doing at another time if he/she is working on a project or playing a computer game as long as he/she stops when the ten minutes are up. We need to recognize that we are asking him/her to do something that is very difficult. Think about how we would react if someone asked us to suddenly stop something we enjoyed immediately.

Fred and Juanita are very frustrated with Vince. He frequently does not follow their directions and often gets angry when they ask him to stop what he is doing. This often results in yelling, spanking, and time-outs. They don't like being angry with him and want to find a better way of handling the situation. They have learned about the five-second rule and ten-minute countdown. Let's hear how it is going from the parents' and Vince's point of view.

Parent Viewpoint

We have just learned about something called "the five-second rule and the ten-minute countdown." We now give Vince five seconds to comply with our directions before we do anything. Supposedly this is the magic time period for Vince to process our direction and start to comply. When he does comply we praise him and if not, he gets a time-out. However, if Vince is in the middle of a game or favorite activity we now give him a ten-minute warning before he is expected to stop.

To our surprise, Vince has started to comply with our directions. Not all of the time, but there is a definite improvement. He also stops what he is doing without a battle when we give him the ten-minute warning. I guess we might have had unrealistic expectations. It really helped to slow things down and give him time to choose to comply with us.

Child Viewpoint

My parents have started counting to five when they ask me to do something. They only ask me twice. If I don't start to do what they want after they count to five, I get a time-out. Most of the time I get myself moving before the count of five. But, if it is worth it, after the count of five, I choose not to cooperate. At least now I have a choice.

When I am doing something fun, like playing a video game, they give me a warning that I will have to stop in ten minutes. They also make sure I can save my video game when I turn it off. I hate having to turn off my computer in the middle of a game. They now give me time to wind down and prepare to stop. Most of the time I can calmly turn off my video game without getting angry.

Summary Parenting Steps

The following is a review of the suggestions made within the chapter of how parents can set their children up for success. They are strategies designed to help parents learn how to teach children new skills, communicate their expectations clearly and visually prompt children to remember daily routines and house rules. The table highlights the strategies noted in the chapter.

- **A. Teaching Is Not a Magic Trick** Break tasks down into manageable segments to help your child to be successful in learning each step.

- **B. Words Are Only as Good as the Visual Images That Accompany Them** Children learn more from what we do not what we say. Modeling is a powerful way in which children learn new behavior.

- **C. Signs in the Right Direction** When you verbally request your child to complete a sequence of tasks, the verbal prompt vaporizes and does not remain as a reminder to your child. A visual reminder, such as a chart, poster, or pictures, is a permanent reminder that can be referred to after the verbal request has been made.

- **D. Say What You Mean and Mean What You Say** Often the child appears non-compliant when the problem really stems from poor communication.

- **E. Posting and Simplifying Rules** Writing a set of simple, clearly written rules and posting them where they cannot be missed increases the likelihood that the child will follow expected rules.

- **F. Five-Second Rule and Ten-Minute Countdown** Research has shown that waiting five seconds before reacting can result in more compliance and avoids unnecessary punishment for non-compliance.

  Giving your child a ten-minute warning with periodic prompts can prevent children from overreacting.

CHAPTER 3

Motivating the Dancers

In the last chapter we learned the basic steps that make dancing with your child easier. Now we are ready to learn how to strengthen the dance, make it fun, and increase enthusiasm for dancing and learning together. You need to learn how to motivate your child if you want your child to choose to dance with you. Once you have used the strategies in the last chapter to make it clear to your child what you want him/her to do, you need to learn strategies to get him/her to do it. Parents cannot make their child do what they want him/her to do if their child does not want to do it. You can only influence the choices your child makes. Learning how to motivate your child to make better behavioral choices is essential to effective parenting.

Positive Reinforcement

Positive reinforcement is a consequence for a behavior and is perceived by your child as pleasurable, and that results in an increase in that behavior over time. The word "consequence" is often associated with punishment, but it is used here to refer to both positive and negative consequences. When a behavior increases in frequency as a result of being followed by positive reinforcement, we say the behavior has been strengthened. Positive reinforcement is unique for each individual. An item or activity can only be determined to be a reinforcer if the behavior it follows increases over time. What one person perceives as positive may not be a positive experience for someone else.

Positive reinforcement does not refer to the intent of the parent in giving a consequence to their child, but rather whether the child's behavior increases in frequency over time when they are consistently given the consequence. For example, you may pat your child on the back each time he/she takes his/her dishes to the sink with the intent of positively reinforcing him/her. If he/she stops taking his/her dishes to the sink over time when you pat him/her on the back, this is not positive reinforcement. If, on the other hand, the child increases taking the dishes to the sink, it is positive reinforcement. You have to try a consequence to see if it is positively reinforcing rather than assuming that it is. Also, we need to appreciate that over time a reinforcer may lose its potency and won't be effective. We may need to change the reinforcer to maintain the behavior.

Timing in the use of positive reinforcement is extremely important. The reinforcer should immediately follow the desired behavior. Whatever the child is doing at the moment you reinforce them, that is the behavior that will increase in frequency. For example, you may be trying to reinforce your child for staying seated at the dinner table. You see your child sitting at the table but get distracted in a conversation. You finally turn to your child and praise him for sitting in his chair when he is actually standing next to his brother. You have inadvertently reinforced him/her for getting out of his/her chair.

Although positive reinforcement works when properly implemented it does not change things overnight. Sometimes people have unrealistic expectations and they get frustrated if there are not immediate and sustained results. However, it may take weeks to months to strengthen a behavior through the use of positive reinforcement. We should not get frustrated, but continue to be consistent, persistent, and patient to effectively apply positive reinforcement in our child's daily life.

What Behaviors Should I Teach?

Deciding on what behaviors to teach your child is important. It should always be made with consideration of what is best for your child. Since you can choose to motivate your child to perform a wide range of behaviors, parents should consider what behaviors will keep your child safe, help them get along with others, and be successful in the settings he/she will encounter.

The materials in the following sections will provide you with a better understanding of the concept and use of positive reinforcement. The materials will also explain how parents can consistently apply various forms of reinforcement to motivate their children. The chapter will be separated into several short sections, which will make it easier to learn and apply. The following briefly identifies the sections that will be discussed:

A. Dances of Love—Understanding Why It Is Necessary to Reward Your Child
B. Leading with Love and Affection—Any Attention Is Better Than None at All
C. Following the Footprints on the Floor—Token of Their Appreciation
D. Leading Naturally—"No Freebies"
E. Dressing Up and Staging the Dance—Packaging

A. Dances of Love—Understanding Why It Is Necessary to Reward Your Child

Parents often feel that they should not have to reward children for appropriate behavior. They believe that children should just learn to behave without parents having to go the extra mile. Sometimes, as parents, we fail to recognize that people, including our children, may need external motivation in order to complete a necessary but difficult task. For example, adults are positively reinforced by the paycheck they receive for going to work. If children help around the house, we need to recognize, or in this case, reinforce them for, their behavior. What may be easy for some children may require a tremendous effort from others. We need to appreciate that some children may need extra encouragement to accomplish what is expected from them.

Scenario 1: Diane and Larry are frustrated with Nick. He will not take responsibility for doing his chores. They constantly remind him and prompt him to get his chores done. They do not feel that they should have to reward him for doing what he is supposed to do. They resist giving him praise and coaxing him because it is against their principles.

They believe that people should be responsible for their own behavior. Let's hear what his parents and Nick are feeling.

Parent Viewpoint

We are at a loss as to how to get Nick to take responsibility for getting his chores done. He doesn't even begin his chores without some kind of a bribe. We constantly battle him and resent having to give him something for doing what he should do without bribes.

Child Viewpoint

I often hear my parents say, "Why do I have to reward you for doing something that you should just do?" I want to know, "Why don't they just do what they should do without a reward?" My mom knows she needs to go on a diet. She knows why she should do this and how people lose weight, but she has to go to Weight Watchers® and have people cheer her on in order to do what she knows she should do. My dad knows he should work out and stay in shape. He shouldn't need someone to tell him to work out or motivate him, but he has a personal trainer that comes to the house every other day. Cleaning my room, doing my homework, doing my chores, and getting my things ready to bring to school each day are things I don't like doing! I need a reward when I do these things.

Solution 1: Dances of Love—Understanding Why It Is Necessary to Reward Your Child

Sometimes we forget what it is like to be a child. We may have unrealistic expectations of children. We forget how difficult it can be to follow simple directions and complete simple tasks. We feel that our children should be able to function independently and not need our constant reminders. We need to get in the world of our children to understand the guidance and support they genuinely need. When we give a direction to follow, we forget that there are competing distractions that are highly important to our children other than what we have asked them to do. Children love to explore their environment and are amazed at the simple things that go on around them. Bugs, flowers, pots and pans, telephones, books, smells, foods, other people playing outside, interesting noises, not to mention TVs, electronics, and computers compete for their attention. Of course, we feel we are the center of the universe and our children should hang on our every word, but reality says otherwise. Considering the range of potential distractions, it is amazing that children ever listen to what we ask them to do. Of course, we are important to our children and they want to please us but receiving recognition in the form of a little motivation seems necessary. Attending to children and recognizing them when they comply with us is a start in motivating children to cooperate with us.

Diane and Larry have decided to try paying attending to Nick when he does his chores. They have also set up a reward for completing his chores. Let's see what they think about rewarding Nick and also see how Nick reacts.

Parent Viewpoint

We were told that bribery is a legal term that means offering a large payoff for doing something illegal. We were definitely not bribing our child. We had to admit that there were times when rewards helped us accomplish a difficult task. It became clear that we were using a different standard for ourselves. When we were faced with a difficult task we often set a goal with rewards for accomplishing the goal. My wife went to Weight Watchers® to lose weight. Each time she weighed in, the group rewarded her. I use a personal trainer to get myself to exercise. We had a double standard. We couldn't discipline ourselves without incentives, but we strongly expected our son to be self-disciplined when faced with a difficult task that wasn't on his priority list. We now no longer resist rewarding our son and are learning new ways of motivating him when he needs it.

Child Viewpoint

Wow, things have changed. My parents are rewarding me and giving me lots of praise. I can even earn special time with them to play games if I do my chores. I now feel good about getting my chores done. Even if the chores are boring, knowing that there is a reward makes doing the chores easier.

B. Leading with Love and Affection—Any Attention Is Better Than None at All

All children want attention, whether positive or negative. If they cannot get attention for appropriate behavior they will try getting it by acting out. In this section, emphasis will be given to help our readers understand that they should positively attend to behavior they want children to exhibit and turn away from and ignore inappropriate behavior that they don't want to occur.

Scenario 2: Sam and Sandy came to us because they were having trouble managing James' behavior. They felt that he was constantly doing things to get their attention. He would act out and do things just to annoy them. They frequently had to intervene to try and redirect him.

Parent Viewpoint

We were extremely frustrated with James. It seems that his behavior is going downhill fast. He rarely listens to what we say. It seems that he is constantly seeking our attention. Nothing we are doing is getting James to do what we ask him to do. He seems to get a lot of our attention when he is misbehaving.

Child Viewpoint

I hardly ever get any positive attention about all the things I do right. In fact, I learned that if I really want attention all I have to do is something they considered to be "bad." I get 100 percent of their attention for anything I do wrong and very little attention for anything I do right. My parents always lecture me about what they expect me to do and when I do what they want, they just ignore me. That isn't fair, don't they realize I need "atta boys" as well? Unfortunately, I have learned a new way to get them to listen to me. I actively seek their attention by thinking up creative ways of being "bad." Let me tell you, this isn't as easy as you think. But if you practice, not only do you get good at it, but also you finally get the attention you are seeking. It works every time. Break a vase, swear, refuse to do what they ask you to do, make loud noises, and try to talk to your parents when they are on the phone. I guarantee you that they will give you their attention. They may yell at you, lecture you, or counsel you, but they will not ignore you. Any attention is better than none at all.

Solution 2: Leading with Love and Affection—Any Attention Is Better Than None at All

Kids are much more observant than parents give them credit for. They are constantly trying to get their parents' attention. Any attention is better than none at all. Whatever a child is doing when he/she experiences something pleasurable is likely to increase the frequency of that behavior. A consequence that increases behavior over time is called a positive reinforcer. What is pleasurable to a child is idiosyncratic and may not be obvious. One way to know for sure is to observe whether the child's behavior increases over time when it is followed by a particular consequence. If a child doesn't get attention for "good" behavior he/she will begin to escalate his/her behavior until he/she gets a reaction.

A child can notice the little things, like when your face turns red or you start tapping your fingers. This tells him/her that you are paying attention. Even yelling and spanking can be a form of attention that he/she may seek if he/she gets little or no attention any other way. The difference is that spanking and yelling makes him/her feel bad, and praise and positive attention make them feel good. Often parents are busy and don't mean to ignore their child, but their child needs some attention to let him/her know that he/she is important to them. We often ignore our child when he/she is "good" and is not causing a problem. Unfortunately we inadvertently pay attention to him/her nearly 100 percent of the time when he/she is behaving poorly. If he/she has learned to get attention by being "bad," it may take a while for him/her to realize things have changed when you try increasing your attention for appropriate behavior. Positive reinforcement takes time to work. It may take several weeks to a month of rewarding your child before there is a significant change in his/her behavior. Don't give up if he/she doesn't respond positively right away.

Sam and Sandy were extremely frustrated. In our work with the family we gave them an exercise called the "Attending Game" with the purpose of trying to explain the concept of positive reinforcement to them. We were trying to get them to realize that if they attended to James when he made an effort to do what they asked, it should lead to an increase in his compliance with them. We asked them to first practice paying attention to any appropriate behavior and then select one behavior, e.g., doing homework, and record what happens. The Attending Game is described below.

ATTENDING GAME

Take twenty pennies and put them in your pocket. Your task is to get the pennies from one pocket to the next. Each time you give positive attention to your child for any appropriate behavior, move one penny to the alternate pocket. Continue attending to your child and moving pennies until you have used up all twenty pennies. Do the best you can at ignoring inappropriate behavior. We will learn alternative ways of responding to inappropriate behavior in a later session on time-out. Do this at least once a day for a week. Note how your child responds to your positive attention.

Now select a behavior that you would like to shape. Think of a problem behavior and what you would like to see your child do instead. Be very clear in exactly what you want your child to do. Starting and continuing to work on homework is a problem for James. Let's focus on attending to James when he is looking at and doing his homework. You may have to verbally prompt James to start his homework if he does not start on his own.

Now take the twenty pennies and move one penny to an alternate pocket each time you attend to James for doing the alternative behavior (doing his homework). Turn away from James and ignore him when he stops doing his homework. Note how your child responds when you increase your positive attention for the targeted behavior. Does James continue to work on his homework for longer periods of time when he is given attention for working on his homework?

Parent Viewpoint

We were surprised to learn that all we had to do to improve the situation was pay attention to James when he was doing what we wanted. We also needed to turn away and ignore him when his behavior was inappropriate. We felt that we were giving him a lot of attention already and this wouldn't make a bit of difference. What we learned was that while we were certainly giving him a lot of attention, it was mostly when he was doing something inappropriate. We never ignored him when he talked back to us, became unbearably loud, or used our computer when we told him it was off limits. On the other hand, we seldom praised him or recognized him in a positive way when he did follow our directions, started his homework, or turned the music down. We realized that from his standpoint, if he wanted attention, he needed to do something "bad." We were given an exercise called the "Attending Game" to try with James. We have to admit that this was hard at first. We were not used to recognizing when James' behavior was "good." This was probably because good behavior was not as obvious as the more extremes of his "bad" behavior.

At first, James looked at us as if he did not trust us. You could see in his facial expressions that he thought we were being weird. This made us aware of how few times we attended to him for "good" behavior. However, we were genuine in our efforts to recognize him for good behavior and he soon accepted our praise and positive attention. We were particularly shocked to see him doing his homework with enthusiasm. In fact, life started to become more fun and enjoyable. Now James seems to enjoy being around us.

Child Viewpoint

I knew that acting up got their attention. We were going along like this for a long time. I had accepted this as being normal. While I was getting the attention I felt I needed the only way I knew how, my parents seemed very frustrated. It worked for me, but it didn't seem to be working for them.

My parents suddenly changed the game plan. I thought we were still operating on the same principle, if you want our attention think of something "bad" to do. Now, suddenly they were lavishing me with praise and giving me lots of attention for everything I did right. I could see that this was not natural and it did not feel natural. At first, I became alarmed. What was happening to my parents? In fact, were these even my parents? It felt so odd. The more they tried to be positive, the more I acted up. After all, I had a system that worked for me, and I wasn't all together sure how this new system was supposed to work or if it would last. I kept trying my old ways and they started not to work. Even though my parents gave me increased positive attention for the "good" things I did, I still occasionally tried getting attention by acting up. After awhile, I began to enjoy the positive attention. I also noticed that it became more natural for my parents. While any attention is better than none at all, positive attention makes me feel much happier.

C. Following the Footprints on the Floor—Token of Their Appreciation

In essence, a token economy is a behavioral approach where parents learn to modify their child's behavior through positive reinforcement. Children learn about acceptable behavior through a system that rewards them with tokens (or stars, points, etc.) on a chart that they can eventually exchange for things they would like to have or activities that they would like to do.

A token system prompts both the parent and the child to consistently focus on specific behaviors. When implementing a token system, parents become more conscious of reinforcing their child for the desired behavior. They are reminded by the token chart to reinforce their child for the behavior listed on the chart. In turn, when their child sees the chart he/she is visually prompted to learn the desired behavior.

Scenario 3: Robbi and Chuck were at their "wit's end." They could not get their son David to comply with anything they asked him to do. They were constantly following him around and asking him multiple times to do his chores and follow the morning routine before going to school. They were angry and frustrated as they described their efforts to gain David's cooperation.

Parent Viewpoint

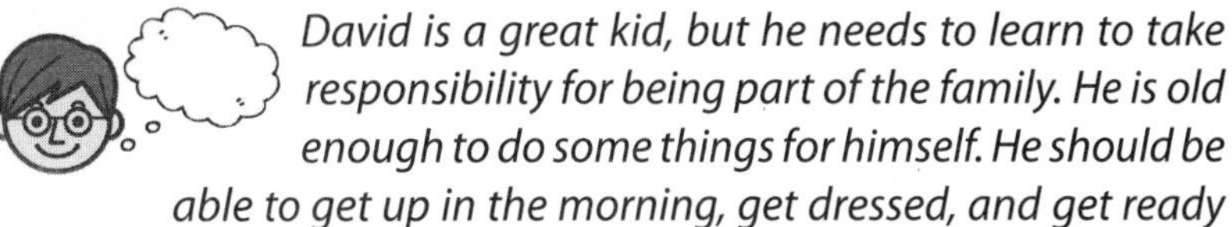

David is a great kid, but he needs to learn to take responsibility for being part of the family. He is old enough to do some things for himself. He should be able to get up in the morning, get dressed, and get ready for school. He should have his backpack ready to take to school each morning without us having to nag him every day. Each morning is a battle. We have to remind David multiple times or he is never ready to leave for school. He always says, "I know" and then ignores us until we end up yelling at him.

Child Viewpoint

My parents are always angry with me. They expect me to be perfect all the time. They are constantly telling me all the things I forget to do and are disappointed in me. I feel sad that they are so upset with me. I try to do the right thing, but I am always getting in trouble. I don't know what to do to make my parents happy.

Solution 3: Following the Footprints on the Floor—Tokens of Their Appreciation

Remembering to pay attention to your child when they do what you want them to do is difficult, but extremely important. A token system helps to remind us of what we expect our child to do and to reinforce him/her if he/she does it. In a token system we recognize our child with a concrete token that could be points, poker chips, stars, marbles in a jar, or anything that you decide to use as a token. The following are the steps to implement an effective token economy.

Steps for Implementing an Effective Token Economy

1. Decide on what you want your child to do. List no more than five or six behaviors. Make sure that you are clear in defining what you want your child to do for each behavior. What would you see them doing? The best way to ensure that your child knows what you mean is to quiz him/her and to role-play. If he/she can give you the correct answer or role-play the answer, then you know that he/she understands.

Parents need to realize that the only reason their child is interested in the token system is because of what he/she can earn. If you only talk about what you need him/her to do, he/she will tune you out. Start by focusing on what he/she can earn and then tell him/her how.

2. Create a chart that both you and your child will enjoy looking at. It could have fun pictures of your child doing each behavior or drawings that your child creates or pictures of his/her favorite cartoon and action heroes.

3. You need to decide how much each behavior on the chart is worth. The more difficult behaviors should be worth more. Make sure you have a behavior on the chart that you know your child can easily earn tokens for accomplishing. This will start him/her off on a positive note and his/her success will increase his/her motivation. Put the value of each behavior on the chart.

4. Post the chart in a prominent place where it can't be missed. The chart will serve to remind your child of the behaviors you expect from him/her and remind you to reinforce him/her each time he/she does them.

5. Decide on what the tokens can buy. You need to spend time deciding on what reinforcers to use. Remember, it has to be something that your child values, not something you *think* they should value. You can determine what might be reinforcing by observing the choices he/she makes when he/she is playing. You can also ask him/her to list favorite items in each area of a reinforcement inventory (see Table 2). However, just because he/she said something was reinforcing doesn't necessarily mean that it is. You have to test using it as a reinforcer and see if your child's behavior increases in frequency over time when you offer it as a reinforcer for a targeted behavior. This is the most

important component of the chart, since it is your child's motivation to respond to the chart. It is important that your child have an opportunity to turn in their tokens daily for the reinforcers. Here is a "Reinforcement Inventory" that you can use to find potential reinforcers:

Table 2
Reinforcement Inventory

List your child's favorite foods:
1.
2.
3.
4.
5.

List your child's favorite drinks:
1.
2.
3.
4.
5.

List your child's favorite things to play with:
1.
2.
3.
4.
5.

List the things your child would like to have:
1.
2.
3.
4.
5.

List your child's friends:
1.

2.
3.
4.
5.

List the places where your child likes to spend time at home:

1.
2.
3.
4.
5.

List the places your child would like to go:

1.
2.
3.
4.
5.

List your child's favorite activities:

1.
2.
3.
4.
5.

List the top ten items in the completed reinforcement inventory.

1.
2.
3.
4.
5.
6.
7.
8.
9.
10.

The items listed in the reinforcement inventory can be made contingent on appropriate behavior.

Once you have a list of potential reinforcers, remember to try them out to see if they are really reinforcing to your child. Children are smart and may try to avoid listing really important reinforcing items because they are afraid you may use them as punishment by taking them away from them when their behavior is inappropriate.

The list of reinforcers that your child can earn should be prominent on the chart. Remember when talking about the chart, start with the reinforcers rather that what you want them to do. This will serve to get their attention.

They should not be able to earn so many tokens that they become millionaires and don't need to behave well in order to turn them in for reinforcers. If your child does not spend the tokens on a daily reinforcer then the tokens should go towards a longer-term reinforcer such as a trip to a favorite destination. It is critical that you review the chart with your child and make sure that he/she understands exactly how the chart works.

Using a token system is an interim step towards a more natural way of getting your child to change behavior. A token system will help you to be clear in what you are expecting your child to do and help you remember to reinforce him/her for doing it. We will learn more natural ways of doing this in the session on "no freebies" and "packaging." Don't get frustrated by the feeling that you are not going to be able to maintain this for a long period of time.

Robbi and Chuck decided to try a token system. What they were doing wasn't working and they were ready to try a new approach. Let's see what happened when they implemented a token system.

Important note: The chart needs to be made child friendly. Children will be more likely to show interest in the chart if they are involved in creating it. Three strategies that can increase children's interest in the chart are:

1. Have your child draw a picture of themselves completing each task for use in the chart.
2. Take pictures of them completing each task for use in the chart.
3. Have them decorate the chart.

	Monday	Tuesday	Wednesday	Thursday	Friday
Get up by 7:00 A.M.	Yes / No	Yes / No	Yes / No	Yes / No	Yes / No
Clean room, take out trash	Yes / No	Yes / No	Yes / No	Yes / No	Yes / No
Get my back-pack ready and leave for school by 9:00 A.M.	Yes / No	Yes / No	Yes / No	Yes / No	Yes / No
Computer time 1 = 15 min 2 = 30 min 3 = 60 min					

Parent Viewpoint

We don't want to reward David for doing what we ask, but nothing else is working. Well, I guess we get paid for working… maybe this is a good lesson for David. Right now, he gets things for free. He doesn't do anything to earn them. We're not giving him money, just privileges. It's free for us, other than putting the chart together and marking it off. David seemed interested when we told him what he could earn and took pictures of him to put on the chart. Getting the point system right turned out to be harder than we thought. First, we gave him too many points, then not enough. We finally got it right. We were shocked when he started doing all the things on his chart. He even reminds us to mark it if we forget.

Child Viewpoint

I just got hired to work for my parents. They gave me a list of things I have to do if I want to get paid in computer time. First they said they overpaid me then they said they underpaid me. Now my pay is apparently just right. I have to get out of bed by 7:00 A.M., clean my room, take the trash out, get my backpack ready, and be ready to leave for school by 9:00 A.M. I can earn one hour of computer time a day. The chart with my jobs is cool. It has my pictures on it. Before the chart, I had to do the jobs for free. Yeah, they had to nag me and even yell at me before I did them, but I didn't earn anything for doing them. Now they don't yell and I don't drag my feet.

D. Leading Naturally—"No Freebies"

Parents often feel challenged in trying to find effective reinforcers to motivate their child. This section will highlight the wide range of potential positive reinforcers that all parents control if they choose to use them. Parents are their child's cook, chauffeur, personal assistant, and provider of all things. Making possessions and privileges contingent on appropriate behavior empowers parents with a wealth of motivators.

Scenario 4: Susan gave her daughter everything she wanted and did everything she could for her. She was upset with how her daughter treated her. Rachel was demanding and rude and expected everything to be done her way. Susan didn't know how to turn Rachel's behavior around or if it could be changed.

Parent's Point of View

I had a very serious problem and was at a loss for what to do. I had exhausted every strategy; I knew and was losing control of Rachel. She felt entitled/ expected everything to be given to her and done for her, even when her behavior was atrocious.

Child's Point of View

My mom is great. She gives me everything I want. She also does things for me. We get along great! Sometimes she says I can't have something I want, but if I really let her know I want it, she gets it for me. Everything is going great!

Solution 4: No Freebies

Parents often have a hard time finding something to use as a reinforcer or motivator for their children. They buy things and offer large incentives such as a trip to an amusement park. When children have everything they want and continue to demand more, parents are at a loss as to what else they can do. The simple answer is "no more freebies." This is also called the "Premack Principle" after David Premack, who first introduced the concept. Premack observed that preferred behaviors could be used to reinforce less preferred behaviors. The Premack Principle is as follows: high-probability behaviors (those performed frequently when given a free choice) can be used to reinforce low-probability behaviors. For example, a parent might make going outside to play (high-probability behavior) contingent on doing the dishes (low-probability behavior).

Parents routinely provide everything for their children free of charge. No matter how children treat them, they chauffeur them everywhere they want to go, prepare their favorite meals, give them unlimited access to TV and computers, and buy them things. Imagine if children had to earn those privileges? Suddenly, you are empowered with an enormous range of motivators right at your fingertips. Children always want to do or have something. Whatever that is at the moment is the most powerful motivator. Even something as routine as helping them to tie their shoes can be a reinforcer. "Mommy, can you help me tie my shoes?" "I would love to help you. As soon as you pick up your toys, I will help you tie your shoes." It is important that you present this in a positive tone. You really want to help them, but first they need to follow your directions. You own everything that your children have and you have a choice in when you help them. Not only does this provide you with a range of natural reinforcers, it also teaches them a valuable life lesson: people are more willing to help you or provide you with privileges if you cooperate with them. If we give things away regardless of our children's behavior, we are teaching them that they are entitled to things even when they treat people poorly. Here is a sample of potential things that can be made contingent on appropriate behavior if children ask for them.

No Freebies

Choice of clothes to wear
Choice of favorite breakfast
Choice of seat in the car
Choice of station on the radio
Choice of route to school
Choice of lunch/dessert
Taxi service (taking your child somewhere they want to go)
Watching TV program
Use of the family computer
Going outside to play
Reading a story at bedtime
Going to a neighbor's house to play
Bedtime
Help with a favorite project
Bringing a friend to the movies
Taking lunch to school in a brown paper bag or a special lunch box
Using a special pen or pencil to write homework assignments

The concept of "No Freebies" can be difficult to embrace for most parents. Parents want their children to be happy and to like them. They have great difficulty in withholding anything from their children because they fear that their children will reject them. We often tell parents that there will be times that they will have to do uncomfortable things that their children won't like. We want our children to love us, but just as importantly, we want them to respect us. We aren't their friends, we are their parents.

Susan was indiscriminately giving Rachel everything she wanted despite her behavior and this led to unintended consequences. Susan became demanding and felt everything should be given to her. No more freebies for Rachel.

Parent Viewpoint

I was helping my child with everything, making her favorite meals and giving her privileges regardless of her behavior. Giving everything away for free was not in Rachel's best interest. I finally decided that "no freebies" was critical and I needed to stick to it. It was a battle of wills between my daughter and me, but I had the advantage. I had all the money, toys, equipment, and property. If she wanted to share in the fun she needed to earn the privilege. I didn't like being the angry, frustrated parent. I wanted my own personality back.

Once I started the no more freebies approach, I felt in control and didn't feel any guilt. Once Rachel got the fact that I wasn't going to give in, she started to get the hang of the concept as well. She was receiving lots of positive attention for good behaviors with rewards and consequences as deserved. No more "freebies." I had everything she wanted, all she had to do was cooperate and enjoy them!

Child Viewpoint

Today my mother told me, "No more freebies". At first I didn't understand that it meant that I no longer got things for free just because I was her daughter. Everything now had to be earned. I was not going to take this lying down. I really believe that I deserve to be given everything I want because that has been the way it has been since I was a baby. There is no reason to change now.

My mom had different plans! I forgot that she controlled everything. She bought all the food, she was the cook, she was my driver, and she bought me my clothes and toys. There wasn't anything that she did not have control of, if she chose not to give me what I wanted, I simply would not get it. It didn't take me long to realize that I was in deep trouble if this was allowed to happen. We were in for a battle. I did everything I could think of to change the game plan. I swore at her and told her that she was a terrible parent who did not love me. I tried to convince her that all my toys and games were mine and I could use them whenever I wanted. My mother saw it differently. She owned everything and if I wanted her help, I needed to cooperate with her. She explained to me that she had not been helping me learn how the world really worked. People don't do things for you unless you cooperate and do things for them. I understood what she was saying but I hated it. Can you imagine going from dictator, having everything you could possibly want, to pauper, having to earn your way? This was a rough lesson. Once I realized that she was committed to the concept of "no freebies" I stopped fighting it and started becoming a pleasant child that my mom wanted to make happy.

E. Dressing Up and Staging the Dance—Packaging

Finding reinforcers to motivate children can be challenging. Parents often run out of ideas on how to motivate their child. They feel that nothing seems to work. However, anything can be made into a powerful motivator by dressing it up with a special name, look, and set of powers that relate to a child's unique interests. We call this "packaging." Parents who learn "packaging" will have an unending source of motivators for their child.

Scenario 5: Joshua was not interested in any of the reinforcers we tried to use to get him to do his homework. We had gone through our entire repertoire of potential motivators and were getting nowhere. If Joshua isn't interested in earning anything we offer him, what can we possibly do? We were at a loss.

Parent Viewpoint

Trying to get Joshua to do his homework was almost impossible. He had a million excuses why he didn't want to do it. He was a master at looking like he was writing when he actually produced nothing. He would promise to do his homework only if we first let him go out and play. He said that he worked so hard at school that he needed a break when he got home. He would forget to bring the books home that he needed to do his homework or tell us that the teacher didn't give him any homework. We tried giving him rewards for doing homework and taking away privileges if he did not do his homework. We were running out of things to give him as a reward and everything we tried did not work. We were running out of ideas. We were desperate to try something new.

Child Viewpoint

I know my parents are really upset with me for not doing my homework. I hate homework. They keep trying to offer me rewards for getting my homework done, but I hate homework more than I want the rewards they give me. I can do without the rewards if it means I don't have to do homework. When I get home I want to play with my friends and forget about school.

Packaging

Parents often feel that nothing can motivate their child to comply with them. They feel that motivation involves giving their children more and more things. Parents feel bankrupt when they run out of things to offer their child. In fact, many things can be made into a powerful reinforcer by how you package it. Marketers make their living by knowing how to package a product. In order to package something as a potential motivator, we have to get into the world of our child and recognize his/her perspective of what is important to him/her.

Many children resist homework. Let's look at how we can take a simple chalk eraser and package it into a powerful motivator for completing homework. Unless your child has a thing about erasing a chalkboard, it is probably not the most motivating object you could use for a reinforcer. Now let's package it so that it is a powerful motivator for your child.

Packaging

1. What can your child do with the eraser if he earns it that will be motivating? Think of what your child might value earning. What privileges would excite him? For example, if he earned the eraser, he could erase a chore, a point loss in his token system, and a loss of privilege.

2. What can we call the eraser to make it more appealing? An eraser is boring. It has no pizazz. What could you name the eraser that would get your child's attention? Are there superheroes that he idolizes? Is there a favorite sports figure he looks up to? The name of the eraser takes on a whole new importance when it reflects something your child values. For example, if your child likes the Terminator we could name the eraser the "Terminator."

3. What will we make the eraser look like? To make the eraser even more valuable to your child, we can morph the eraser into the "Terminator." We can put a picture of the Terminator on the eraser or have your child draw a picture on paper attached around the eraser.

4. How will we talk about it, or build it up? *"We have something special that we are going to tell you about tomorrow. It will give you special powers to eliminate chores, and point losses in your token system. You are really going to like this."* Now we can use earning the "Terminator" as a reinforcer or reward. Using this same process, you can make anything reinforcing.

Bob and Mary can't get Joshua to do his homework. He was a master at avoiding homework. They had tried giving him rewards when he attempted his homework and taking TV time away from Joshua when he didn't do his homework. They felt that they had exhausted their use of rewards and nothing seemed to get his attention. They did not know what to do to get Joshua to do his homework. We gave them the example of using an eraser as a reinforcer for completing homework. They doubted it would work but they decided to try actually "packaging" an eraser and using it to motivate Joshua to do his homework.

Parent Viewpoint

We were very skeptical that we could make an eraser into a powerful motivator. We decided to try the packaging concept. First, we had to determine what the eraser could do that would be important to Joshua. We decided that it could erase a chore or a loss of minutes of TV. We knew this would get his attention. We then gave a special name to the eraser to make it more interesting to Joshua. We decided to call it the "Terminator" since Joshua would like that name and it was named after his favorite action figure. We even glued a picture of the Terminator onto the eraser.

The next step was the build-up to introducing the "Terminator" to Joshua. We sat Joshua down and told him that we had a very special thing we wanted to show him that he would really like. We told him that we were going to show him the object in the next couple of days. This seemed a little cruel because Joshua was excited by the possibility of getting something special. He kept asking us all day long what we got for him. After two days, we showed him the eraser. His face dropped and he asked if we were joking. We told him that we weren't joking. He said, "That's an eraser, what's the big deal?" We responded by saying, "It is not an eraser, it is the 'Terminator!'" We asked if he wanted to know what he could do with the "Terminator." He said, "Duh, erase a blackboard." We quickly told him that we knew it could erase things, but it could also do much more if he earned it. It could erase a chore or a loss of "TV time." He suddenly became interested and asked, "What do I have to do to earn the 'Terminator?' "You have to start your homework and show us that it is complete." Much to our amazement, David started doing his homework to earn the "Terminator." We were surprised to learn that even an eraser could be a powerful positive reinforcer. We started "packaging" other things, and even made a special homework area we called his "Executive Office."

Child Viewpoint

My parents said that they were going to introduce a new fun thing for me to earn in a couple of days. I was busting at the seams to know what they got for me. Next, they pulled out an eraser dressed up as a superhero. They told me that it was the "Terminator." Wow, what do they think, I'm supposed to get excited about an eraser masquerading as a superhero? I was about to tune them out when they asked me, "What do you think you can do with the 'Terminator' if you earn it?" I sarcastically said, "Erase the blackboard." They then explained the unexpected. It could erase much more. Like magic it could erase a chore or even a loss of minutes of TV for "bad" behavior. Now that got my attention. I said, "What's the catch?" They said, "No catch, just an opportunity to erase something of your choice if you earn it." I decided that they could "package" all they wanted if I got something fun out of it. My homework area suddenly became my personal executive office, dinner had a different theme each week, and I was excited.

Summary Parenting Steps

As parents we often find ourselves trying numerous alternatives to get our children to follow our directions. Unfortunately, our children don't come with a manual and at times their behavior tests our limits. Some parents find themselves becoming frustrated and applying negative alternatives. We believe that constructive alternatives such as positive reinforcement are critical to meet the challenges. If our children are to attempt new and challenging tasks, they may need encouragement and support from us to make the change. Reinforcements will help motivate our children to persist in their efforts.

The use of positive reinforcement has several beneficial effects. Applying properly implemented reinforcers helps parents support and guide their children as they successfully adapt in their lives. Applying reinforcers correctly helps parents create a positive bond between themselves and their children. It also helps to create a healthy environment, which indirectly impacts their child's well-being and sense of healthy self-esteem. Focusing on how to positively reinforce and encourage your children will allow you to more comfortably interact with your child without conflict.

Applying reinforcements may seem simple and truly can be, when following accurate guidelines. We believe that to be effective in applying positive reinforcements, we need to get into the world of our children and truly understand their interests, likes, and dislikes. Without being able to accurately identify your child's unique interests, we as parents cannot apply proper reinforcements that will work effectively. When expertly applied, it will make a world of difference not only in your role as a parent, but also in the manner in which your child will respond to you.

A. Dances of Love—Understanding Why It Is Necessary to Reward Your Child
Sometimes, as parents, we fail to recognize that people, including our children, may need external motivation in order to complete a necessary but difficult task. What may be easy for some children may require a tremendous effort from others. We need to appreciate that some children may need extra encouragement to accomplish what is expected from them.

B. Leading with Love and Affection—Any Attention Is Better Than None at All
All children want attention, whether positive or negative. If they cannot get attention for appropriate behavior, they will try getting it by acting out.

C. Following the Footprints on the Floor—Token of Their Appreciation
A token economy is a behavioral approach where parents learn to modify their child's behavior through positive reinforcement. Children learn about acceptable behavior through a system that rewards them with tokens (or stars, points, etc.) that they can eventually exchange for things they would like to have or do.

D. Leading Naturally—"No Freebies"
Parents often feel challenged in trying to find effective reinforcers to motivate their child. Parents control a wide range of potential positive reinforcers if they choose to use them. Making possessions and privileges contingent on appropriate behavior empowers parents with a wealth of motivators.

E. Dressing Up and Staging the Dance—Packaging

Finding reinforcers to motivate children can be challenging. Many parents feel that nothing seems to motivate their child. However, anything can be made into a powerful motivator by dressing it up with a special name, look, and set of powers that relate to a child's unique interests.

CHAPTER 4

No Time for Tap Dancing—Let's Tango: Steps to Decrease Non-Compliance and Opposition

The previous chapter focused on the importance of motivating children to make more appropriate behavioral choices. When children are more motivated to behave appropriately, there may be fewer incidences of inappropriate behaviors. However, when they act out or engage in dangerous behavior, parents need strategies to quickly and effectively stop those behaviors. In this chapter, parents will learn how to effectively respond when children act out or put themselves in harm's way. We will focus on some very basic, but potent strategies, such as ignoring, time-out, and an approach called "Response Cost," to decrease inappropriate behavior.

Ignoring is completely removing all attention to a specific behavior with the goal of decreasing the behavior. Response cost and time-out are forms of punishment. Punishment is the presentation of a consequence for a specific behavior that results in a decrease in that behavior. Response cost is the removal of points in a token system, privileges or a favorite possession, or a fine for a specific behavior that results in a decrease in that behavior. Time-out is the temporary removal of all reinforcement for a specific behavior. Fact Sheet 1, Guidelines for the Use of Punishment, is provided at the end of the chapter. The difference between punishment and reinforcement is simple. Punishment decreases or weakens behaviors while reinforcement strengthens the behavior.

Parents will learn how to effectively stop minor inappropriate behaviors, such as making verbally annoying noises or tapping objects, by ignoring these behaviors. They will also learn strategies to decrease or stop dangerous, oppositional, or socially inappropriate behaviors through the use of response cost and time-out. Ignoring, time-out, and response cost are effective ways of stopping children's inappropriate behavior. While the use of these strategies may sound easy, it can often be undermined. Parents will gain insight into the potential pitfalls in using ignoring, time-out, and response cost.

The following chapter will be separated into four sections, which will focus on these basic strategies designed to decrease or stop misbehavior:

How to React When Your Toes Get Stepped On:
A. Ignoring
B. Response Cost
C. Time-Out
D. The Art of Crying and Fussing

A. Ignoring

Sometimes children do things that are irritating to us. They may not do these things intentionally, but they are hard to ignore. If we give them attention for these behaviors, they may become worse. One choice is to completely ignore the behavior. If the child does not get attention for the behavior, it may slowly begin to decrease or stop altogether. Ignoring a new annoying behavior is one option for stopping a minor problem behavior.

Scenario 1: Larry and Janet are beginning to dread having dinner with Keisha, their daughter. When they are having dinner she starts tapping her spoon on the table or plate. They ask her to stop, but she keeps doing it. They don't know why she is doing this, but it is starting to get worse. Keisha is beginning to really annoy them.

Parent Viewpoint

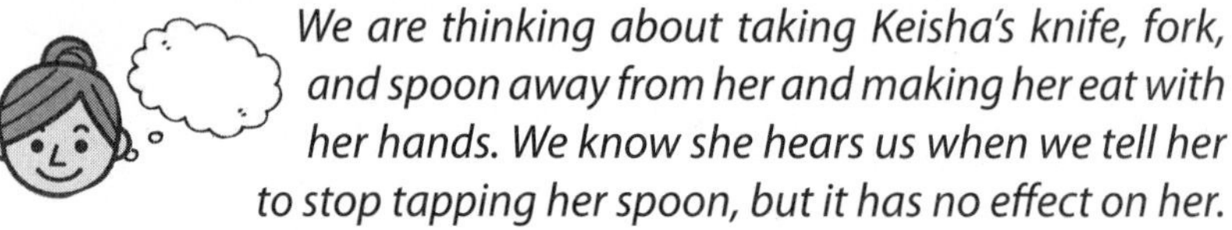

We are thinking about taking Keisha's knife, fork, and spoon away from her and making her eat with her hands. We know she hears us when we tell her to stop tapping her spoon, but it has no effect on her. Telling her to stop tapping her spoon is only making it worse. It's like she enjoys annoying us.

Child Viewpoint

Wow, what's the big deal! So I tap my spoon, it's fun. My parents make angry faces that look really funny and make me want to tap more.

Solution 1: Ignoring

Often parents say, "He/she is just trying to get our attention." In fact, this may actually be the case. Even if your child did not start out trying to get your attention, he/she may inadvertently make the connection that his/her behavior is increasing your attention to him/her. One strategy that may decrease an annoying behavior is ignoring.

There are several considerations in deciding to use this strategy. Is this behavior dangerous? You cannot ignore dangerous behavior such as running in the street. Is this a behavior you can realistically ignore? Children are very astute at recognizing any reaction you may have to their behavior. If you turn red with embarrassment, make a facial expression as a reaction to the behavior, or laugh, they know you are attending to them. This can be enough to increase the behavior. Are there other people in the setting that will react to your child, even if you are not? This will undermine the effect of ignoring since your child can still get attention for his/her behavior.

Ignoring may not be a good choice if your child has been occasionally getting attention for bad behavior for a long period of time. Compare it to winning at the slot machine occasionally: you keep playing because you just might win on the next try.

Ignoring is a strategy that works best with a new behavior. It is important to realize that the behavior might get worse before it gets better. At first, your child will increase the behavior before he/she realizes that you are not going to respond to it. Slowly, over time, the behavior will begin to stop.

Larry and Janet realize that Keisha's behavior is not extreme, but it is beginning to annoy them. They do not want to overact, but they need a way of getting Keisha to stop tapping her spoon on the table or plate. They have calmly asked her to stop, but she is tapping her spoon even more. They are going to try completely ignoring her when she taps her spoon to see if this will get her to stop.

Parent Viewpoint

You should see Keisha's face. We totally ignored her when she tapped her spoon at the dinner table. She looked puzzled. She kept trying to get us to react and even tapped her spoon louder. We could see her slowly giving up. To our surprise she stopped banging her spoon after only one week of ignoring.

Child Viewpoint

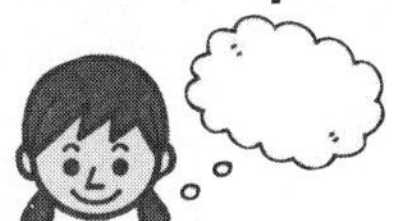

Wow, my parents seem to have lost their hearing. I keep tapping my spoon louder and they act like nothing is happening. They're taking the fun out of it.

B. Response Cost

Response cost is an efficient form of punishment that can be used to decrease inappropriate behavior. As stated previously, punishment is the presentation of a negative consequence for a specific behavior that results in a decrease in that behavior. Response cost is the removal of points in a token system, privileges, or a favorite possession, or a fine for a specific behavior that results in a decrease in that behavior.

Scenario 2: Celine and David are very busy. Their son, Charlie, drags his feet whenever they are in a hurry to get somewhere. This often makes

them late. They are beginning to think he enjoys stirring things up and seeing them rush around frantically waiting for him.

Parent Viewpoint

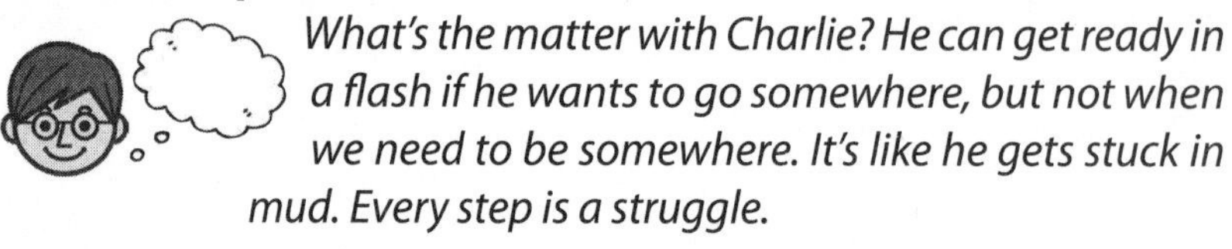

What's the matter with Charlie? He can get ready in a flash if he wants to go somewhere, but not when we need to be somewhere. It's like he gets stuck in mud. Every step is a struggle.

Child Viewpoint

I just want to stay home and play. They always tell me they don't have anyone to watch me and I have to come with them. I don't need anyone to watch me. Why do they always want me to go with them? It's boring.

Solution 2: Response Cost

As stated above, response cost is a form of punishment in which points in a token system, privileges, or a favorite possession are taken away for a specific inappropriate behavior, which results in a decrease in that behavior. Response cost can also be a fine for a specific behavior. If you are using a token system and want to use response cost to help decrease inappropriate behavior, you have to decide how many points in the token system you will take away. You should take enough points to have an impact without bankrupting your child. For example, if he/she can earn fifty points a day, taking sixty points each time the behavior occurs will result in your child giving up. "*Why should I keep trying, I'll never earn enough points to earn anything*?" Taking ten points for each incidence of the behavior will still give him/her enough points to earn something in his/her token system, if he/she stops the behavior, and get his/her attention without bankrupting him/her.

If you are taking a privilege or possession away, you need to decide what privilege or possession you will choose. You can create a hierarchy of a most valued to least valued privilege or possession. You also need to make sure that your child cannot play with the possession at someone else's house, or go around you in getting the privileges somewhere else. As with points in a token system, you do not want to bankrupt your child by increasing the consequences and continuing to take more and more possessions and privileges away. Once you take all of their possessions and privileges away, you have nothing left to use. You also do not want to take a favorite possession or special privilege away for long periods of time. If you take a toy or privilege away for a week, you no longer have a powerful consequence to use during that week. Your child might as well go for it. They have nothing to lose. It is best to take a privilege or possession away for no more than a day. If their behavior has been good for the rest of the day, they can get the possession or privilege back.

Celine and David are beginning to miss important appointments. They try to find someone to take care of Charlie so he doesn't have to go with them to appointments, but on occasion they don't have anyone to watch him. Charlie drags his feet in protest and makes them late for appointments. They are going to try response cost to get Charlie moving.

Parent Viewpoint

Charlie suddenly freed himself from the mud and gets ready to go with us without a struggle. It only took three days of losing ten minutes of computer time for each minute he took getting to the car. All we have to do now is say, "That's ten minutes," and he hustles to the car.

Child Viewpoint

Man, my parents are serious about me coming with them! I can't believe they are fining me ten minutes of computer time for every minute I am late to the car. I don't have my own computer. I only get one hour a day to use my parent's computer. I have to admit, I was enjoying the ruckus I was causing. Not anymore!

C. Time-Out

"*I hate you. I don't want to go to the store with you.*" How often have you heard these words? Often, we find ourselves overreacting to a child's defiance rather than staying calm and not overreacting. We need to apply strategies that will help us to stop dangerous, oppositional, or socially inappropriate behaviors. We cannot be ruled by opposition, but must teach our children to conform to reasonable guidelines. Time-out has been found to be an excellent strategy to stop children's inappropriate behavior. While the use of time-out may sound easy, it can often be anything but. We will demonstrate the problems parents can expect when they first try using time-out and how to avoid them.

Scenario 1: John and Irene came to us for advice on how to handle Mark's rude and aggressive behavior. They had tried sitting Mark down and lecturing him about his misbehavior. They told Mark that they expected him to treat them and others with respect and that they would not tolerate his rudeness. Unfortunately, talking and lecturing didn't have any impact. This led to their frustration, which resulted in them yelling and spanking him. The price was high, but it temporarily stopped the behavior. The rudeness returned. John and Irene needed a more effective way of responding to Mark.

Parent Viewpoint

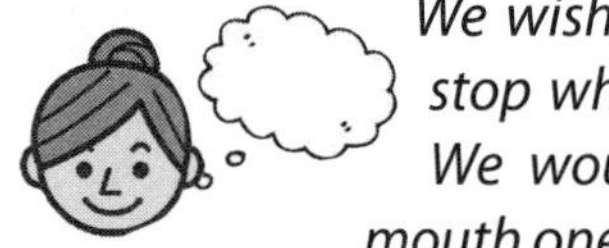

We wish we could wave a wand and get Mark to stop what he is doing! Wow, he is so headstrong. We would love to tell him that if he opens his mouth one more time, we would cast a spell over him. Too bad we don't have that magic wand that will make that change. Mark knows that, and we feel powerless. We are not proud of yelling, but that seems to be the only thing that gets his attention

Child Viewpoint

My parents sure get mad at me. Unless I am rude or do something that they don't like, I rarely get their attention. I know it seems strange, but I like

it when they both sit down with me and give me a lecture. I have their undivided attention. I hear what they are saying, but I like all the attention I get when I talk back to them.

Solution 1: Time-Out

Don't Just Teach What Not to Do Without also Teaching What to Do

Time-out is a form of punishment in which all reinforcement is temporarily removed from the child for a specific behavior. The use of punishment, such as time-out, only tells a child what not to do. If the behavior that is reinforced is the exact opposite of the problem behavior, you may not need to use punishment. Whenever you use punishment for an inappropriate behavior, you need to also reinforce your child for an alternative appropriate way of responding. If the behavior that is reinforced is the exact opposite of the problem behavior, this may solve the problem. You may not need to use punishment. For example, when your child is constantly getting up from the dinner table, positively reinforcing him for staying in his/her chair may solve the problem. Staying seated in the chair is incompatible with getting up from his/her chair. If a child uses a rude and demanding tone to ask for what he/she wants, effective punishment should stop the behavior. However, if he/she is not taught an alternative way of asking for what he/she wants, he/she will continue to be rude. This is technically known as positively reinforcing incompatible behavior.

However, there are times where this may not work. You could positively reinforce your child for talking nicely to his brother as an alternative to saying mean things. He/she may increase positive statements to his/her brother but still say mean things when you aren't around. Positively reinforcing him/her for saying nice things to his/her brother will increase the incidents of him/her saying more kind words, but it may not stop the problem behavior entirely. Unfortunately, positively reinforcing a child for incompatible behavior does not always entirely stop the undesirable behavior, so other options will need to be explored.

Time-Out

Time-out is the temporary removal of all reinforcement for a specific behavior. Most people don't realize that time-out actually means time away from being reinforced. It is important that the environment from which the child is temporarily being removed be reinforcing to the child. The time-out environment must be considered less appealing than the environment the child is presently in. The time-out area must be boring and away from the action. You cannot be reinforced when you are asked to sit in a place that is boring and completely devoid of any attention. If the time-out area is actually more enjoyable, it may defeat the purpose.

There are several things that parents must consider when utilizing time-out.

Time-Out Steps

1. When giving a time-out, you must remain calm. This does not imply that you are totally calm, only that you make your best effort to calm yourself and not be reactive. If you raise your voice or become agitated, it may escalate the problem.

2. You need to be very clear about what behaviors will result in a time-out. Some behaviors automatically result in time-out. These are behaviors that we cannot tolerate because they are dangerous, destructive, or extremely socially unacceptable. This category may include acts of aggression, destroying property, or rudeness to others. The second category is repeated non-compliance. Compliance for children can be considered a safety factor. For example, if a parent says, "stop running," when the child is about to enter the street in front of an oncoming car, a parent needs to know the child will stop. Not everything that you ask a child falls into the category of safety. But, if a child has not generally learned to comply with a parent's voice command, it is highly unlikely that he/she will comply when it is critical.

3. Parents have to decide how many times they are going to give their child a direction before giving them a time-out. A child will learn the exact number that a parent is using by the number of times the parent typically repeats himself/herself before finally following through with a time-out. The goal is to have your child follow your direction after one request. We believe that two requests are sufficient. Parents should give a child five seconds to respond between each request. If a child does not comply after the second request he/she has earned a time-out.

4. Once a parent gives a child a direction to go to time-out, the parent should not get into a discussion about anything that he/

she says. Everything the parent says and does should be aimed at getting him/her to do the time-out. A child will naturally try to get out of doing a time-out by making you feel guilty or changing the subject. Here are some typical statements that children may say when you when you ask them to go to time-out.

"I hate you."
"It's your fault that that I have a time-out."
"You're stupid."
"Why do I have a time-out, I didn't do anything?"
"You have a time-out."
"You don't love me."
"I won't do that again, do I have to have a time-out?"

Once you tell a child they have a time-out, do not respond to any of these statements. Simply repeat the direction to go to time-out. A parent can make an empathetic response, but needs to follow through and make sure the time-out is delivered. For example, a parent might say, "I know that you are angry, but you still have a time-out." The empathetic statement can serve to defuse your child's anger.

5. Now that we know what behaviors result in a time-out, we need to decide where the child will go for the time-out. Designate a time-out area that is boring and away from the action. For example, a designated chair can be put in a hallway or an area of the house that is seldom the focus of activity. If we are in a public area, we need to decide where best to do time-out. Find an area that is away from others and is as boring as possible. This adds a special challenge of following through with an audience. If you plan ahead on where you can successfully do a time-out in public, you will feel less self-conscious.

6. Parents need to decide how long time-out will last. It is better to use a short time-out. Most people suggest no longer than one minute per year of age. That would mean that a five-year-old's time-out would be for five minutes. The time-out may be extended for longer periods when the child continues acting out in time-out and has not sat quietly for the designated time period.

7. We then need to explain to the child exactly what is expected from him/her when taking a time-out. For example, while sitting

in time-out, the child should sit quietly and remain seated until released from time-out. To ensure that the child understands what is expected, you can role-play taking a time-out.

8. Remember that time-out is the punishment. We should not lecture the child about the behavior or hold a grudge. Also, we should not try to extract a confession. This may result in the child escalating into another time-out. We also do not want to counsel the child immediately after a time-out. Counseling can be viewed by the child as a very pleasant experience. Your child may try to get in time-out just to get the counseling.
9. Once the time-out is over, give him/her a direction of what you want him/her to do after taking a time-out. For example, "*John, your time-out is over, you now have a direction to pick up your toys.*" Once the child's behavior has been "good" for a period of time, remember to start praising him/her for "good" behavior.
10. You need to decide what backup consequence your child will get if he/she refuses to go to time-out or leaves early. The backup consequence is response cost as an added penalty. For example, if a child refuses to go to time-out he/she could lose TV time, a favorite toy, computer time, playing with a friend, or anything else of value to the child.

Table 1 is an easy-to-follow Time-Out Script. The script is designed to help parents know exactly what to say and do when giving a time-out. Fact Sheet 2, Planning Ahead, is also provided in the back of the chapter to help parents problem-solve if time-out does not seem to be working. Here in Table 1 is a script for giving time-out:

Table 1

Time-Out Script

TIME-OUT SCRIPT

Behaviors that result in a direction to go to time-out: Aggression, destruction of property, rudeness, and non-compliance.

"You _______________, (hit someone, kicked someone, were rude to someone, destroyed something), you have a direction to go to time-out."

Releasing the child from time-out:
"Time-out is over, you have a direction to ________________(tell him/her what you want him/her to do)."

Script for repeated non-compliance.

First request: "You have a direction to Pick up your toys please."

Count to five before giving the second direction.

Second request: "You have a direction to *pick up your toys or you will have a time-out.*"

Count to five before giving the third direction.

If he/she follows your direction to pick up his/her toys, praise him/her for following your direction. If not, give him/her a time-out.

Third request: "You are choosing not to follow my direction, you have a time-out."

At this point he/she must do the time-out before he/she does anything else. "The only time-out that didn't work is the one you didn't do."

If he/she does not choose to go to time-out then you tell him/her that he/she will be given a backup consequence:

Fourth request: "You are choosing not to follow my direction to go to time-out. You will be losing _______________ (minutes of TV time, computer time, a favorite toy, etc.)

John and Irene are frustrated with Mark's rude behavior. They have decided to try using time-out to stop Mark's rude behavior and reinforce him for using socially appropriate language.

Parent Viewpoint

We explained to Mark how time-out was going to work. At first, Mark was defiant and refused to go to time-out. He told us he hated us, we were mean, and we couldn't make him go to time-out. This derailed us at first, but we realized that all his huffing and puffing was an attempt to get out of doing time-out. Once we added response cost, he seemed to get that we meant business. After a week of losing TV time for not going to time-out, he started to respond more favorably. When told to go to time-out, he did. Apparently, he did not want to lose TV time.

Next, we ran into an unexpected problem. Mark seemed to be trying to get into time-out. Because of our guilt over punishing Mark, we reassured him of our love immediately after he completed time-out. We finally realized that we were inadvertently reinforcing Mark for getting a time-out. It took three weeks before time-out finally started to work again.

Child Viewpoint

When my parents told me about time-out my reaction was, "Right! You are going to get me to sit in a boring area for a few minutes each time I am bad, not likely." If I try hard I can get things back to the way they were. "Bring it on." I told them, "No, I'm not going and I don't care what you do." They told me if I didn't go to time-out I was going to lose TV time. I really did not want to lose my favorite TV show even though I said I didn't care. I didn't cooperate at first, but they held their ground. I missed my favorite program four days in a row. On the fifth day, I was a believer.

This worked for them for quite a while until one day I realized that when my parents released me from time-out they immediately told me that they loved me and what a wonderful child I was. What I noticed, though, was that I never got this level of affection when I was "good," only after I was given a time-out. I began looking forward to getting a time-out. Yes, I did think it was strange that I had to sit for a short period of time away from them in order to get their unconditional love, but what the heck, this was working for me.

One day they suddenly changed. I kept expecting the love after my time-out and all I got was a neutral response. I also eventually noticed that I didn't need to get myself into a time-out to get unconditional love. In fact, my parents seemed to notice when I was doing "good things" and stopped to give me praise, hugs, and kisses. It took me a while to catch on that things had changed. Also, I learned that there was no real advantage to getting myself in a time-out.

Before my parents learned how to use time-out they were yelling at me, spanking me, and putting me down. Yelling, spanking, and verbally putting me down made me feel terrible. Time-out tells me what not to do without making me feel bad about myself. I don't like to get a time-out but it does not affect my self-esteem.

D. The Art of Crying and Fussing

Parents often become trapped in a cycle of giving in to their children's demands. Children learn early to whine, cry, and nag until they get what they want. Parents learn that in order to stop the whining, crying, and nagging, all they have to do is give in to the demands. Crying and fussing as an infant may turn to whining and nagging as an older child and even as an adult. We will learn how to avoid this cycle and help our children learn more appropriate ways of getting their needs met. We need to alter this way of approaching things and show children that nagging and whining won't work. Let's look at an example of how crying and fussing can generate negative responses.

Scenario 2: Tim and Sharon are frustrated that Linda constantly cries and nags them to get what she wants. She is three years old and should have outgrown these alternatives. Her parents are diligently trying to get Linda to use her words instead of fussing when she wants something. She seems resistant to change because it has worked for years.

Parent Viewpoint

I hate this!!! What was expected when she was a baby is no longer cute. We didn't mind her crying then, because we knew it was her only way of communicating her needs. Now at three years old, the amount of crying is off the charts. We don't dare deny her anything because she will wake the neighborhood with her loud crying and complaining. We believe that the only to way stop her annoying nagging and crying is to give in to her. We don't like giving in to her but we don't know what to do.

Child Viewpoint

Life started off pretty great. All I needed to do was to cry or fuss and everything came to me. If I was hungry, I fussed and I got fed. If I was cold, I fussed and I got a warm blanket. If I was wet, I fussed and my clothes were changed. If I just wanted to be picked up, all I had to do was fuss and then cry. I was the master of my universe. Everything I needed and wanted was provided at my every whim. What a life! My parents didn't always know exactly what I wanted, but they learned through trial and error. My parents taught me an important lesson, cry and fuss and I could get what I wanted NOW.

Solution 2: The Art of Crying and Fussing

We dance our first dance with our children at their birth. We are attentive to all of their needs in order to keep them safe and comfortable. Over time, we become aware of all of their movements and behavioral quirks. Some of us will become capable of deciphering and decoding the various sounds in their crying and fussing and will be able to differentiate their meaning (e.g., telling us they need their diaper changed, are hungry, cold, hurt, or just want attention). In essence, our infants cry or fuss until we figure out what they want. When we "get it," they stop.

When our children are infants we are more accepting of their whining, crying, and fussing because we understand that is how they communicate.

However, as they age, this option of communication becomes less tolerated. Our children must learn more developmentally acceptable approaches of getting their needs met. Using language is the greatest tool for this change. Once infants develop to the point where they can use their words, they need to learn that their old reliable approaches (e.g., crying and fussing) are not going to be accepted.

This is easy to understand when we think of people who nag and bully until they get what they want. Most of us don't like associating with this type of person and it is only natural we do not want our children to have these qualities as well. Once children are able to clearly express themselves with words, we must teach them more suitable ways of getting their needs met. Whining, fussing, and crying should now be ignored and our children must be encouraged to use appropriate words to get what they need. When we choose to respond to inappropriate reactions, we indirectly reward their behavior and encourage more negative responses.

Since we have described parenting as a dance, we need to look at the "art of crying and fussing" from the child's viewpoint. In this way, we can better understand the power of this negative cycle. Tim and Sharon are ready to teach Linda to use her words instead of crying and nagging to get her way. Let's look at the first dance, "The Art of Crying and Fussing."

Parent Viewpoint

Linda is now three years old, capable of asking for something when she wants it. We don't want to create a monster. No one will want to be around her. We both know adults who whine and nag to get their way. We avoid them. We don't want this to happen to our daughter.

Not giving in to Linda is a real battle. She yells, cries, and constantly nags to try and get what she wants. She even gets louder to wear us down. The only way this can work is if both of us support one another. We prompt her to use her words and walk away when she whines and nags. We are now even giving her short time-outs. This seems to be working and the whining is slowly decreasing. We praise her, and make sure she is successful in getting what she wants when she uses her words. She is slowly learning to use her words to get what she wants. Linda gets a time-out when she whines or nags and praise when she uses her words. Our patience and consistency has paid off.

Child Viewpoint

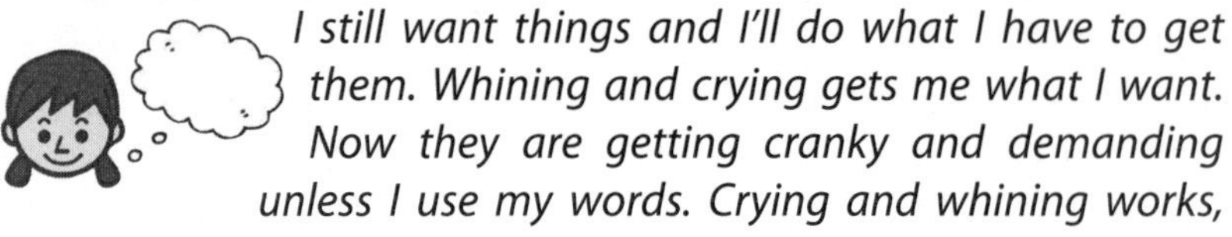

I still want things and I'll do what I have to get them. Whining and crying gets me what I want. Now they are getting cranky and demanding unless I use my words. Crying and whining works, why change now?

I am ready for a battle. I am determined to keep things the way they have always been. Well guess what? For weeks, we had a see-saw battle. Sometimes I won and they gave in while other times, they stuck to their guns. They made me use my words. I hate having to use words. It is easier to fuss! Our battles were exhausting for both of us. In the end, I held out for three weeks. They let me cry and whine for hours and just ignored me. They also started giving me time-outs! They even stopped giving me what I wanted until I used my words. I was hoarse from yelling and screaming. I finally began to use my words and then they would cooperate with me. Well, I gave up my pacifier last year, so I guess getting older comes with a whole bunch of changes.

Summary Parenting Steps

In this chapter we learned strategies for stopping inappropriate or dangerous behaviors. Once a dangerous or inappropriate behavior is stopped we need to teach our children an alternative appropriate behavior. Punishment only teaches a child what not to do but does not teach them what to do instead. The following is a summary of the parenting steps learned.

A. Ignoring

Ignoring is a strategy that can be used to decrease or stop a minor annoying behavior. Ignoring a behavior means giving absolutely no attention to the behavior. We do not ignore dangerous behavior. Ignoring is also not a choice if the behavior cannot realistically be ignored because it produces a strong emotional response. The parent is unable to control their response to the behavior. Ignoring will also not work if someone else is attending to the behavior. Finally, it will take a long time to decrease the behavior through ignoring if, in the past, the behavior has been reinforced occasionally.

B. Response Cost

Response cost is a form of punishment in which the child loses a favorite toy, points in a token system, or privileges for a specific behavior. The loss of a toy or privilege needs to be for a brief period of time. Parents should not continue to take multiple things away or they will bankrupt themselves and the child. The child will feel that they have nothing left to lose and might as well go for it. Parents will also lose the use of these favorite toys or privileges as a consequence the next time the behavior occurs.

C. Time-Out

Time-out is a form of punishment in which the child is removed to a boring area, away from all positive reinforcement, for a specific problem behavior. Time-out is for a short period of time based on the age of the child, one minute for each year.

D. The Art of Crying and Fussing

Who would have imagined that we could get so easily trapped into a cycle of giving in to our child's aversive demands? In this section we highlighted how children learn that nagging will get them what they want. Unfortunately, we have taught them this by giving into their whims when they were quite young. We now have learned that it is critical to not get sucked into a child's fussing, but to teach the child that he/she cannot always get his/her way. Also, we need to show our child that he/she must use words to tell us what they need and to realize that "yes" isn't the only answer we can give.

Fact Sheet 1

Punishment Guidelines

Punishment Guidelines

A. Individualized for each person

The choice of punishers should be based on a punishment inventory that is specific to your child's likes and dislikes. What is a punishment to one child may actually serve to reinforce another child.

B. Should be immediately following the behavior

What ever your child is doing when you punish him/her is what is actually being punished. If you delay punishment, you may actually be punishing desired behavior. If your child is playing nicely with their sibling and you finally get around to giving them a time-out for what he/she did twenty minutes ago, you are in fact punishing him/her for playing nicely with their sibling. Timing is critical.

C. Should be something in your control

If you have taken away Nintendo as a punishment and they go next door and play Nintendo, then your punishment has been undermined. Make sure that you can follow through with any consequence that you may choose to use.

D. Should be done in a calm manner

Try to remain calm when punishing your child. If you raise your voice or become emotional, you may escalate the problem. Your choice of punishment (time-out, loss of privileges, etc.) is the only punishment needed. Yelling only serves to escalate your child's behavior. Once your child is responding with a great deal of emotion, they are not processing what you are saying and doing.

E. Should be explained to the child in advance

Your child should know exactly what is expected of him/her and what the punishment will be if he/she violates your rules. He/she should also know exactly what you are expecting him/her to do when he/she gets punished. For example, if you are using time-out, he/she should know exactly what your expectations are for taking a time-out appropriately. If you let him/her know in advance, he/she will be less likely to feel the punishment is unfair and escalate his/her behavior. You are merely following through with what you had told him/her you would do.

F. Should not be for a long period of time (hours, days, weeks)

Punishment should not be extended for long periods of time. If you make the punishment for long periods of time, your child will have no reason to turn his/her behavior around. You also are continuing to punish him/her when his/her behavior may now be exemplary. You bankrupt yourself. For example, if you take a privilege or toy away from him/her for a week, you no longer have this as an option if the behavior occurs again within the week. If this is your most powerful consequence, you have handicapped yourself. Also, if your child feels that his/her punishment will continue for a week, he/she might as well continue the inappropriate behavior.

G. Should not be followed immediately by counseling

Oftentimes parents feel guilty about the use of punishment and immediately begin to counsel their child. If this pattern develops, your child will learn that if he/she wants counseling all he/she has to do is act out. To avoid this connection, counseling should follow appropriate behavior. Wait for a period of time in which your child has been demonstrating appropriate behavior following a punishment such as time-out. Counseling is now associated with appropriate behavior.

H. Should not try to extract a confession or statement of remorse

Your child has done the time. Extracting a confession or statement of remorse may escalate the behavior again. If you were clear about your expectations and the consequences for the choices your child makes, it is not necessary to have him/her state what he/she has done.

I. Should be followed by reinforcement after a period of time in which the child is complying with you and has demonstrated appropriate behavior

After your child has been given a punishment such as time-out, you should begin to reinforce your child for appropriate alternative behavior. Remember to allow a period of time immediately following the punishment so that you child does not learn that the only way they can get reinforcement is to first be punished.

J. Should only focus on stating what the child needs to do to complete the consequences, and not unrelated topics

Children will try all kinds of tactics to avoid punishment. Don't get sidetracked by engaging in conversations that have nothing to do with the punishing consequences.

Remember, you are punishing the child for making inappropriate choices, not because he/she is bad. Everyone makes mistakes. You are helping him/her to realize that certain choices will result in punishment. You do not want to give him/her the message that he/she is a bad child.

Fact Sheet 2

Planning Ahead

Did I clearly state what behaviors would result in an automatic time out?

Second, did I explain what time-out behaviors will include a warning such as repeatedly not following directions?

Did I explain where my child would be taking time-out?
(Did I select a time-out area with no competing distractions or reinforcers?)

Where will my child take time-out: at home, at a restaurant, at a relative's house, or in the car?

Did I explain how long time-out would be?

Did I explain the rules of appropriately taking a time-out? What would taking a time-out perfectly look like?

Did I explain what happens if my child does not take a time-out appropriately or resists? What would the backup consequence be for not taking a time-out?

Examples of backup consequences:
Loss of Privileges:

1. Make a hierarchy of privileges from most important to your child to least important.
2. Make sure that you can follow through in taking away the privilege once you state that your child has lost the privilege.
3. Decide on how long your child will lose the privilege. Remember, if you take the privilege away for a long period of time you will lose this consequence in the near future. The consequences should be given immediately and last for a relatively short period of time.
4. Let your child know what he/she needs to do to regain the privilege.
5. Remain calm when informing your child that he/she has lost a privilege so he/she does not become emotional and escalate his/her behavior.
6. Do not get talked out of following through. It is important that your child learns that you say what you mean and you mean what you say.

Loss of a Favorite Toy or Game:

1. Make a hierarchy of favorite toys or games.
2. Make sure that if you take a game or toy away, they cannot get another one from a neighbor.
3. Do not continue to take more and more toys and games away in sequence if your child continues to be non-compliant. You will bankrupt yourself.

4. Take toys and games away for a relatively short period of time, long enough to be effective but not for days and days. In addition, if you continue to punish over long periods of time, you are forcing yourself to punish your child even if their behavior has improved and is exemplary.
5. Don't give in and give the toy or game back after telling him/her they have lost it for a period of time. Say what you mean and mean what you say.

What type of punishment would be practical to use in the following situations? (Choices: time-out, loss of a privilege, and loss of a favorite toy or game)

In a market:
In the car:
At home without visitors:
At home with visitors:
In a park:
In a restaurant:
At someone else's house:
At your parents' or relatives' house:

Did I stay calm when giving a time-out or backup consequences?

My plan for tuning up my time-out:

CHAPTER 5

Avoiding Missteps

In the Parent-Child Dance there are many opportunities for missteps in parenting. Within this chapter we will focus on some potential missteps and discuss practical solutions to avoid these errors. Missteps in the Parent-Child Dance lead to unfortunate sidetracks that prevent parents from implementing parenting strategies successfully.

For example, in some instances, a child may attempt to split parents so that they can get what they want. If they don't hear what they want to hear from one parent, they sneak off to ask the other parent. As a result, the parents do not present a united front. The child can choose to align with the parent who agrees with them.

Parents often find it difficult and embarrassing to parent their child in public. They ignore their child's behaviors and let the behaviors escalate until they can no longer be ignored. At this point, their parenting is overactive and emotional. The child learns that in public there are few, if any, rules.

Another challenge is when your child is with others and not directly under your supervision, such as school, or at a neighbor's house. A child may act very differently at school or with a neighbor than they do at home. This presents a unique challenge. How do parents extend their influence over their child to settings where they are not present?

How we are feeling affects how we assess the effectiveness of our parenting. It is natural to have good and bad days. When we are feeling bad we see everything in a negative light. If someone asks us how things are going with our child we may say, "Terribly." In fact, if an objective observer were watching how our child was actually doing, he/she may disagree. Our child may be doing well, but we have a hard time seeing that when we don't feel well. In order not to get derailed we need to recognize the role of our emotions in our assessment of our parenting or we may give up on an approach to parenting that is actually working. This is true for our child as well. They have good days and bad days. It may be that our child just doesn't feel well and is acting out. The question to ask ourselves in assessing whether our parenting strategies are working is: "Am I having more good days or bad days?" If in the long run we are having more good days, then the strategies are working. Our child just had a bad day.

Parents may choose not to use effective parenting strategies because they are too busy. They know what to do but don't do it. If parents don't use the strategies they learn, they will not benefit their child. Finally, parents are not given a manual on how to parent their child. In Table 3, a card with prompts of the parenting strategies learned in the previous chapters is provided for parents to refer to as a reminder of what choices they have in parenting their child. The following sections give some basic suggestions for avoiding missteps:

A. Always Dance with the One You Came With: Divide and Conquer
B. Dancing with an Audience: Don't Change the Steps When Performing in Public
C. Learning to Dance with Others: Out of Sight, Out of Mind
D. Good Days and Bad Days
E. A Special Case of the "Yeah, Buts"
F. Owners' Manual

A. Always Dance with the One You Came With: Divide and Conquer

It is important that parents present a unified front and understand how they can avoid being split by their child. A child may often try to split their parents by going to the parent who will give them the answer they want to hear. By splitting parents, they can always get what they want.

Scenario 1: Lately we feel that our daughter is playing Parent Ping-Pong. She goes between the both of us fishing for the answer she wants

to hear. If she doesn't like the answer that her mother gives her, she slyly goes to me to see if I will give her the answer she wants. This creates fights between us because each parent feels undermined by the other. As we argue, Ellie goes off to do what she wants, since one of us told her she could do it. It's hard to catch her doing this, because she always asks us when we are busy and in a hurry. I think she has this down to a science.

Parent Viewpoint

Wow, how did we get in this situation! Ellie is a master manipulator. She knows how to get the answer she wants. My wife and I rarely agree on anything and this has spilled over into our parenting. Until we find a way to work together, Ellie rules the roost.

Child Viewpoint

My parents always argue. I hate it, but it works for me. I ask to do something and throw the question out. One of my parents will side with me. When I hear what I want, I smile and hug the parent who agreed with me. I leave them to argue and go off to do what I want.

Solution 1: Always Dance with the One You Came With: Divide and Conquer

Learning to dance is difficult and confusing if more than one person is giving you directions. What if the advice is conflicting: To whom do you listen? In the Parent-Child Dance, conflicting directions between parents have the same effect. Children become confused and uncertain as what to do. Your child is uncertain as to who is in control. They now have an option to choose whom to listen to. The natural choice is the one that is in their best interest. "I like what Dad said, I think I will follow his direction." We call this "splitting parents." We have all heard the saying, "divide and conquer." Well this is what is happening. The child is aligning with one parent against the other. They have a perfect defense: "That's what Dad said" or "That's what Mom said." This can lead to arguments between parents. Your child is free to do as he/she pleases while their parents hash out who is "right."

Parents don't always agree, but your child does not need to know this. Disagreements can occur in private and consensus reached without your child knowing. It is important that you support one another in front of your child, and if there is a disagreement, discuss it in private. A child cannot split parents who support one another. Remember, it is normal to have differing opinions but not constructive to argue in front of your child.

Dennis and Susan came to us for help because they couldn't agree on the best way to parent Ellie. It seemed that they were always arguing. This was especially true when it came to parenting Ellie. This became clear when each parent tried to gain our support for his or her point of view. Both parents stated their case and then looked to us for support. When we asked them if they did this in front of Ellie, they had to admit that they did.

We told them that the problem was not who was "right" and who was "wrong," but how they resolved the problem. Effective parenting requires parents to be consistent and supportive of one another. They need to present a united front. If they argue in front of their child, the child is forced to choose between parents. The child is most likely going to choose to follow the direction of the parent who is going to allow them to do what they want. Both parents felt it was unrealistic for them to agree on everything, including how to parent Ellie. We told them that we agreed with them and that the problem was in how they resolved the disagreement.

First, they needed to agree not to argue in front of Ellie. Second, they needed to agree to support one another in front of her. They could agree to disagree, just not in front of Ellie. Third, they needed to set time aside to reach consensus in private when there was a disagreement. Once one parent gives an instruction, the other parent needs to support that parent even if they disagree. In private they can then discuss their concerns and reach consensus on how the problem will be handled in the future. Let's see how this worked for Dennis and Susan.

Parent Viewpoint

It took all our self-control not to contradict one another. I had to bite my tongue to keep from arguing in front of Ellie. We still argue, but in private. We have some long debates, but Ellie never sees them.

With a smile, we support each other. If Ellie tells me that her mother said it was all right to do something, I say, "If I ask your mother will she tell me it's okay with her?" I then check with Sue to see what she said. Ellie slowly stopped her Parent Ping-Pong. To our surprise, the private meetings to discuss how to parent Ellie spilled over and now we are beginning to compromise on other issues. An unintended benefit is that we are getting along better.

Child Viewpoint

My parents have finally caught on to what I was doing. I didn't consciously set out to split my parents to get what I wanted. It just worked out that way. One day I went to my dad after my mom told me I could not go out and play. When I asked my dad he said, "Sure you can go out and play." Worked for me. It wasn't until they began fighting that they realized what I was doing. I can still catch them once in a while, but it rarely pays off. They ask me, "If I ask you father, what would he say?" I know better than to lie because they now check with one another. They call this splitting parents. If I split my parents, I get an automatic time-out.

B. Dancing with an Audience: Don't Change the Steps When Performing in Public

Perhaps one of the greatest challenges for some parents is when they find themselves parenting in a public setting. Parents are often embarrassed by their children's behavior and are hesitant to follow through with consequences in a public setting. Some parents find it awkward to discipline their children in a public setting, especially when their children are non-compliant. This eventually compounds the problem. Children often learn that parents have one set of rules when they are at home and a second set of rules in public. Children indirectly learn that rules don't seem to apply in public settings. This section will help to foster a better awareness of parenting in a public setting. Within this section, viable solutions will be proposed, making parenting in public environments easier to put into place.

Scenario 2: Lee is flabbergasted by Susan's behavior in public. At home she is an angel and rarely causes any problems for Lee. In public, she transforms into a monster. There is no relationship between her behavior at home and in public. Lee sometimes pretends that Susan is not his child when she starts her antics.

Parent Viewpoint

That's It! I'm not taking Susan out of the house. As soon as she crosses the doorway and has an audience, she turns into a monster. She starts talking back to me, wanders off, doesn't listen to me, and gets into everything.

Child Viewpoint

As soon as we leave the house and we go somewhere, my dad changes. It's like he's waiting for me to do something wrong. I can't help getting excited and exploring all the fun things around me. I start running everywhere and I guess I get loud. My dad ignores me like he doesn't know me. It always ends with him getting angry and taking me home.

Solution 2: Dancing with an Audience: Don't Change the Steps When Performing in Public

Rehearsing and performing a dance is difficult enough without the stress of an audience. With an audience we are self-conscious and concerned with how we appear as we perform the dance. The Parent-Child Dance in our home can also be difficult and stressful. Once we master the dance at home, we must choreograph it for public performance. We must also master our fears and prepare ourselves to handle the challenge of parenting in public. For example, we may know exactly where we will send our child to time-out at home, but where should we do time-out at the restaurant? There are many things for our child to do at home when there is downtime, but what can they do when waiting for food at a restaurant? If we become increasingly embarrassed by our child's behavior in public, we may start to avoid going out to public places with him/her.

One way to desensitize ourselves is to practice when we don't have anything else we have to do. For example, we can go to a market with our child when we don't need anything from the market. We can develop a plan with our child and go to the market with the sole purpose of practicing how to behave in a market. Since we don't need anything, we are free to attend to our child and it will be easier to follow through with the plan we developed. We can also try this in a mall or any public place we would like to be able to take our child. Like dancing, parents in the Parent-Child Dance can only become comfortable performing in public by doing it. Here is a form for use in planning ahead for an outing:

THE PLAN!

Preparing for an Activity

Excursion to:

Goal of excursion:

Anticipated problems:

Plan to solve anticipated problems:

The specific rules of this outing:

Strategies to increase behavior

Behaviors I will PRAISE:

Behaviors I will GIVE TOKENS for:

Token to be given:

Behaviors I will use "NO FREEBIES" for:

Strategies to decrease behavior

Behaviors I will IGNORE:

Behaviors I will REDIRECT:

Behaviors I will give a TIME-OUT for:

Time-Out Location:

Time-Out Length:

Backup consequences if my child is refusing to take time-out:

Behaviors that will result in LOSS OF PRIVILEGE:

Possible privileges to take away:

Now that we have developed a plan, it is important that we review the plan with our child before the activity and several times during the week. The goal is to practice preparing our child for an activity to increase the probability of his/her success. Often we develop a plan for an activity without making sure that our child is aware of our expectations. Taking the time to brief our child will save us many potential hours of frustration. The following are suggested steps in preparing our child for an activity:

1. Pick a time when your child is relaxed and ready to communicate with you. Using the "no freebies" rule can help to motivate your child to participate in planning for an activity. "First we're going to discuss going to the store and then you can go out and play."

Time: ______________________________

Place: ______________________________

No freebies rule:

"First we're going to discuss ____________ and then we can __
________________________."

Potential freebies:
a. ____________________________
b. ____________________________
c. ____________________________
d. ____________________________
e. ____________________________
f. ____________________________

2. Explain your plan in a simple and concise manner. To make sure that your child understands what you are explaining, probe them for understanding. Make sure that you praise your child for attempting to answer your questions. You can also ask questions in the form of a game. "I'm going to test you on what I just explained and you can earn a penny for every correct answer." If you are still not sure that your child understands what you are expecting or whether they have the skill to do what you are asking, you can role-play with them. Make sure to ask your child if they have any questions about your expectations. If they have suggestions that you can incorporate, then add them to your plan. If your child comes up with ways to handle situations, he/she will have more buy-in to the plan.

Lee has been working for several months on his home program. Things have been going well, and he is finally feeling confident in his ability to parent Susan. However, in public "all bets were off." Lee does not seem to have any control. He no longer goes out in public with Susan unless he absolutely has to. Going to the store, a restaurant, or the mall is a nightmare. Sometimes he even pretends Susan isn't his child.

It is clear that in public Lee is embarrassed and extremely emotional when Susan acts out. He does not seem to be learning from his past outings. He does not take the time to plan how he is going to respond to Susan's behavior in public. Susan's behavior in public is predictable. Lee can tell us exactly what she will do but not how he will react.

Lee needs to address two problems. First, he needs to draw on what he learned in developing his home program. He needs to have a plan before going out in public. Second, he needs to be desensitized to parenting in public. Lee practiced making a plan to go to the market when he didn't need anything. Susan and Lee went to the market to practice the plan. After three similar trips to the market, Lee became more confident. Let's see how Lee and Susan feel when there is a plan in place.

Parent Viewpoint

I couldn't believe how quickly Susan changed her behavior when we went to the market with a plan. It helped that I didn't need anything from the market. Of course, she didn't know that. You should have seen Susan's face the first time I gave her a time-out in the market.

Having a plan for going to the mall and a restaurant worked just as well. Now I feel more confident and relaxed when we're in a public place. I like taking Susan with me.

Child Viewpoint

How weird! Dad sat me down and said, "Let's plan going to the market." Why … we never did this before? Why do we need a plan to go to the market? Dad told me that if I followed the plan I could buy something at the market that I wanted. He also told me I would get a time-out if I didn't follow his directions. He even told me where the time-out would be. He shocked me and I felt embarrassed when he actually gave me a time-out in the market. I will never do that again. Now we go lots of places, but with a plan.

C. Learning to Dance with Others: Out of Sight, Out of Mind

Often a child may act differently when their parents are not present. Parents are surprised to hear teachers, friends, relatives, and others describe their child's behavior when they are not around. In this section parents will learn how to extend their influence to settings outside the home.

Scenario 3: I was shocked to hear how Ron was behaving at school. He didn't act anything like that at home. The teacher called me and asked

me what I was going to do about Ron's behavior at school. I was stymied. How can I do anything about Ron's behavior when I'm not there?

Parent Viewpoint

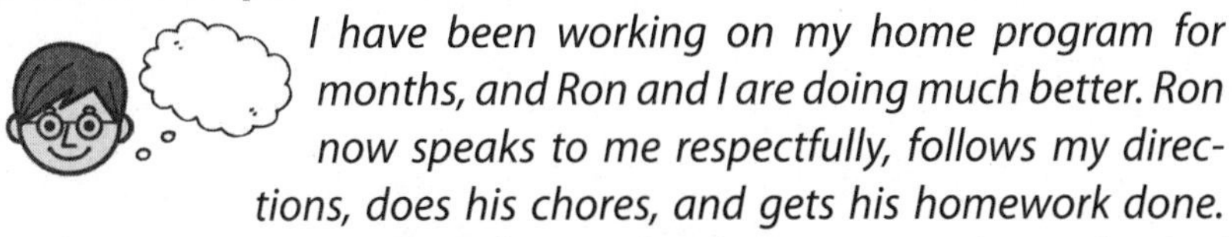

I have been working on my home program for months, and Ron and I are doing much better. Ron now speaks to me respectfully, follows my directions, does his chores, and gets his homework done. Today I got a request from his teacher for a meeting. I was shocked to learn in the meeting that Ron was getting into fights, was rude to the teacher, and didn't do his work in class. He was even sent to the office on several occasions. The teacher had been trying to handle the situation on her own and had finally had it. She wanted to know what I was going to do. I was stymied. What could I do? I wasn't at school and I couldn't go to school with him daily. When I got home I sat Ron down and lectured him about the importance of listening to his teacher. I threatened to ground him for a month if he kept this up and made him write one hundred times "I will be good at school." He said he was sorry and it wouldn't happen again. Unfortunately, he didn't keep his word any more than I did. I didn't ground him for a month. I finally decided I needed to try something different.

Child Viewpoint

Everything is going well at home. The one time that I am free to do as I like is when I am out of my dad's sight. When I am at school, at a friend's, at the church class, or anywhere Dad is not there to watch, I can do as I please. Sometimes I do what I used to do at home before Dad started the new rules. At school I get myself in trouble just to avoid having to do school work. My teacher sends me to the office. In the office I have a great time watching everything that goes on and I don't have to do work. At my friend's house, I often get in trouble because I argue with my friend Bob's parents and get wound up and loud when playing with Bob. His parents don't know what to do to get me to stop. Sometimes they just send me home. At church school, I get bored and try to get myself kicked out of class. I am having a great time at my friend's house and I have learned some great ways to get kicked out of class but my teacher seems to be losing her temper with my antics.

Solution 3: Learning to Dance with Others: Out of Sight, Out of Mind
Once parents have perfected the Parent-Child Dance at home and in public, the challenge is how to extend parenting to other settings such as school or a neighbor's house. "Out of sight, out of mind." Even when "in sight," children often don't always comply. The question then is, "How do I get my child to behave when I'm not there?" The answer is a "Daily Report Card (DRC)." This is an extended token system that goes with your child to the next setting, for example, a neighbor's house, school, or Little League practice. The DRC is a simple report card with the expected behaviors listed on it.

To extend your influence over your child's behavior, you need to meet with whoever is supervising your child and identify the behaviors that are causing problems in that setting. Their role will be to go over the DRC with your child and give him/her feedback at regular intervals of what they've earned on the DRC.

The first step in developing the DRC is to decide what you want your child to do, instead of the problem behavior. Usually this will be two or three behaviors. Find out how often these behaviors occur. Next, determine realistically how often your child will need feedback to maintain their positive behavior. You want to try and reinforce your child on the DRC frequently enough to avoid the problem behavior from occurring. Unless the supervisor agrees to more intervals, there should be no more than three intervals. Most people will agree to three checkpoints. If your child is going to be at your neighbor's house for three hours, your child could be given feedback each hour. The supervisor meets with your child in private and reviews the target behaviors on the DRC. He/she then marks whether they met the goal or not. The DRC goes home with the child, and the parent reviews it with him/her. Depending on his/her performance on the DRC, he/she can earn several levels of reinforcement.

You want to avoid an all-or-none system because as soon as your child loses the opportunity to earn some reinforcement, they will give up. If there are three problem behaviors and the supervisor marks the report card three times, there is a possible nine points the child can earn. You can break the levels of reinforcement into three levels: 7–9 points, 4–7 points, 0–4 points. As an example, the child might earn staying up forty-five minutes later at night if they earn 7–9 pts., thirty minutes if they earn 4–7 pts., and normal bedtime if they earn less than 4 pts. The DRC gives you the opportunity to bridge your home program with other settings.

Carl was completely shocked to hear how Ron, his son, behaved at school. At home, Ron was polite, followed Carl's directions, and even did his chores without reminders. You can imagine how disappointed he was to hear that Ron often got into fights with his peers, was rude to the teacher, and disturbed the classroom when he was supposed to be working independently. Carl met with the teacher and she asked Carl what he was going to do about this.

Carl decided to try setting up a DRC with the teacher. This would require collaboration between the teacher and Carl through a Daily Report Card (DRC). The teacher could fill out the DRC and send it home each day with Ron. Carl could provide the motivation to do well on the DRC and cooperate with the teacher.

The first step was to meet with the teacher to learn exactly what Ron was doing that was causing a problem. Once it was clear what Ron was doing wrong, Carl needed to learn what Ron should be doing instead. What would Carl see Ron doing in the classroom if he was doing what the teacher wanted? In Ron's case he needed to: 1. Keep his hands and feet to himself and speak respectfully to his peers, 2. Follow the teacher's direction with no more than one reminder, and 3. Complete the assigned work. These behaviors were written on Ron's DRC.

The next question was how often Ron would get feedback on his DRC. The teacher agreed to give Ron feedback three times a day: before recess, before lunch, and when he left for home. The teacher agreed to meet privately with Ron and briefly state whether Ron met the behavioral goal on each behavior and mark the DRC accordingly. Ron could earn a potential of 9 pts. each day. The teacher signed the DRC validating the score each day. Carl's responsibility was to greet Ron each afternoon, review the DRC, and reinforce Ron if he earned enough points. Carl had completed a reinforcement inventory and decided computer time was the most powerful reinforcer for Ron. Carl and the teacher decided that they should not use an all-or-nothing approach. Depending on the number of points Ron earned, he could increase his minutes of computer time. If Ron earned 7–9 pts., he earned one hour of computer time, if he earned 4–6 pts., he earned thirty minutes of computer time. If he earned fewer than 4 pts., he earned no computer time. Let's hear how Ron and Carl feel about the DRC.

Important note: The chart needs to be made child friendly. Children will be more likely to show interest in the chart if they are involved in creating it. Three strategies that can increase children's interest in the chart are:

1. Have your child draw a picture of themselves completing each task for use in the chart.
2. Take pictures of them completing each task for use in the chart.
3. Have them decorate the chart.

Ron's DRC

Ron's Report Card	**First Recess**	**Lunch Recess**	**End of Day**
Keep your hands and feet to yourself	Yes / No	Yes / No	Yes / No
Follow the teacher's direction	Yes / No	Yes / No	Yes / No
Complete the assigned task	Yes / No	Yes / No	Yes / No
Total Points:			
Reward	9–7 One hour computer time	6–4 Half hour computer time	Below 4 No computer time

Parent Viewpoint

I needed a way of extending my control over Ron to the classroom. Since I couldn't be there, I needed a way to monitor Ron and consistently motivate him to comply with his teacher. We agreed that Ron would be monitored through the use of a Daily Report Card that went home daily. The teacher would mark the card and I would reinforce Ron based on his performance.

The DRC was working well with the exception of the days Ron decided not to bring it home. On those days he said he earned all his points. I learned that actually he hadn't earned enough points for computer time. We made another rule: if he did not bring his report card home he automatically lost computer time.

The DRC turned out to be a great tool for any situation in which someone else was supervising Ron. Now Ron can go to a neighbor's, Little League practice, or camp, and I can use the DRC to influence his behavior.

Child Viewpoint

I can't believe the teacher ratted me out to my dad. School has nothing to do with my dad. The teacher and my dad ganged up on me. They started a report card that goes home. My computer time is no longer free. If I don't do well on my report card I lose computer time. What a bummer! My dad did the same thing when I went to my friend Bob's house and with the church school. The long arm of the law was now following me everywhere I went. While I resented the report card at first, it helped me have a better time with Bob, and fewer problems with my teachers at school and church.

D. Good Days and Bad Days

Parenting can be exhaustive when we consider everything we have to do in a day. If we allow ourselves to get run down and exhausted, we may not be able to objectively evaluate how our children are doing. We may not be able to see our children's progress. We need to take care of ourselves if we are going to be able to take care of our children.

It is also important that parents realize that it is normal for children to occasionally have bad days. A bad day does not mean that the parent's home program is not working. Parents need to look at their children's behavior over time to evaluate how effective their parenting is.

Scenario 4: Nothing seems to be working. I feel so tired. I don't have the energy to do anything. I've tried to do everything I was taught to help Rick and to no avail. I am ready to give up. Here is what Ruth and Rick are feeling.

Parent Viewpoint

Nothing is working. I feel like I am back to square one. I frankly don't have the energy to keep trying. Why can't Rick just do what he's supposed to do without all the drama? I love Rick but I need a vacation or I am going to get sick. Maybe if I could get some rest things would seem better. I don't know if Rick is really getting worse or I just feel that way because of how tired I am?

Child Viewpoint

Today I heard my mom say, "Nothing is working. We're back to square one. Why can't he just be good without me having to work so hard all the time?" I have been doing everything she asks me to do. Today I just had a bad day. Give me a break. Most of the time I am in a good mood and cooperate with my mom. What's the big deal that I don't feel warm and fuzzy on occasion? If you asked me, I wouldn't be able to tell you why I feel funky. Maybe I am coming down with a cold, or something happened that made me feel bad. I guess it just happens.

When Mom has a bad day, she translates it to me. She sees me through her funky glasses and I can do nothing right. I have learned to recognize when she is having a bad day and try to avoid her. Why can't she accept me having a bad day? This was beginning to become a real problem. My mom panicked and started to do things the "old way." She started yelling at me again.

Solution 4: Good Days and Bad Days

It's hard to dance well when we don't feel well. Even though we know how to do the dance and have been dancing well, when we feel tired and exhausted the dance doesn't go well. It's natural to have days when we just don't feel like dancing. As a dancer, we know the show must go on. There will be other days where we will feel better, and as a result, dancing will come easier.

In the Parent-Child Dance there may be times when we feel we don't want to parent. We just don't feel up to it. This is not a choice, and we know we still need to parent. When we feel better, our parenting will be more effective. This is also natural and as parents we need to recognize this and accept that this will happen. To avoid "bad" days, we need to take care of ourselves. We need to go to the doctor when we are sick, and seek respite when we are tired and run down. When we don't feel well, this is not the time to assess whether our parenting strategies are working or effective. Invariably, when we feel bad the answer will be "no." Whether our parenting strategies are effective needs to be assessed over time. If our child's behavior has improved over time then the answer is "yes" and our parenting strategies are working.

The same is true for our children. They can have "bad" days as well. For example, something may have happened at school that we are unaware of, like a fight with a friend. On that day their behavior is difficult. They are having a tough time letting go of the fight. It has nothing to do with you. Children have "good" days and "bad" days just like their parents, and we need to recognize this as normal and not change how we parent. We can empathize with their feelings but not change our parenting. For example, we may say, "I know you are upset, but you hit your sister, and you have a time-out." You are recognizing his/her feelings but still holding him/her responsible for his/her behavior.

Ruth came to us with the complaint that nothing was working with Rick. Ruth looked tired, worn out, and angry. As we quizzed her about what was happening with Rick, we learned that actually his behavior had gotten better. Although Ruth stated nothing was working and she was frustrated, when we probed further, we learned that Rick's behavior was actually improving. Before Ruth started her home program, Rick never did his homework. Now Rick completed his homework on most days. Rick seldom cleaned his room before Ruth started a token system to get Rick to clean his room, and now he was cleaning his room. It soon became clear that Ruth was discounting her successes because she was assessing Rick through the fog of her exhaustion. She could not see things in a positive light because she felt so bad. We suggested that she take time for herself. She needed some downtime to rest and gain the strength to parent. We suggested that she have Rick stay with a relative while she took time to rest and do something fun for herself. She needed to put her feelings about how effective she was as a parent on hold. Once she had rested, she could revisit her feelings about her home program.

Parent Viewpoint

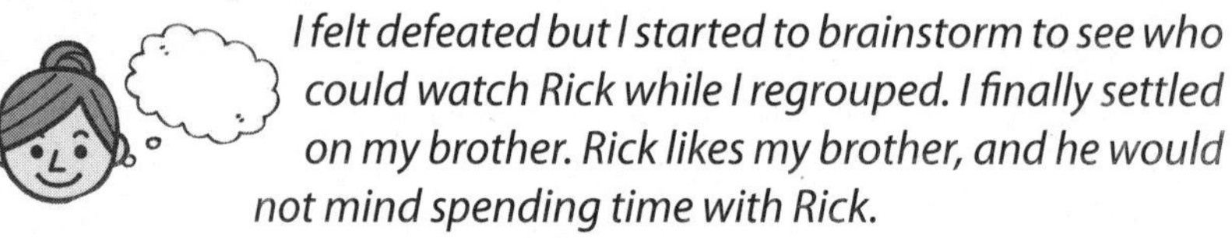

I felt defeated but I started to brainstorm to see who could watch Rick while I regrouped. I finally settled on my brother. Rick likes my brother, and he would not mind spending time with Rick.

I arranged for Rick to go with my brother and finally had time to myself. I slept in and read a novel I had wanted to read. I went for walks on the beach and saw several movies. I began to feel better and started to miss Rick. I had my brother bring Rick home. We were both excited to see one another again.

A surprising thing happened. Even though I did not change anything I was doing, I started to feel good about how things were going at home. I realized that nothing had changed except me. I was rested and feeling happier. It is amazing how just a little time off had re-energized me. I'm committed to taking time for myself anytime I start to get tired and down. I am doing this as much for Rick as I am for myself.

Child Viewpoint

My mom looked tired and angry all the time. Suddenly, she said she was going to take time for herself and sent me to my uncle's for a week. I like my uncle and we have fun. When I came home from my uncle's, I noticed that my mother's behavior had changed. She now stayed calm and even started to recognize how I was feeling, saying things like, "I see you are upset, but you still have to do your homework," when she saw I wasn't feeling well. When I hear her say these words I know that she understands that I am having a "bad day" and I try harder. I can also see that when my mother is rested and feels good, things go much better.

E. A Special Case of the "Yeah, Buts"

Parenting is the most important thing we will ever do, but not the only thing we have to do. We have many tasks in a day that interfere with effective parenting choices. Some choices we make in parenting our child may not be effective because we don't know what to do. Other times we know what to do but we choose not to do it. We call this the "**yeah, buts**." "**Yeah,** I know I should have followed through with a time-out **but** I needed to go to the store." "**Yeah,** I know I should have started homework earlier in the day **but** I didn't want to miss the Angels game." The good news is that when parents reach the stage of "**yeah, but**" they know what to do. The bad news is that if they know what to do but find excuses not to do it, they will not benefit from what they know. If we don't use effective parenting strategies, things won't go well. At this point the goal is not to learn new strategies but to eliminate the "**yeah, buts**." If we are unaware that we are doing this we can't change it. We have provided a form for parents to use in recognizing when they are using "**yeah, but**," as an excuse for not doing what they know they should. Each time we find our self saying or thinking "**yeah, but**" we need to write it down and develop a plan to avoid it in the future.

Yeah, But

I know I should have ______________________ but:

I know I should have	But	Plan to eliminate the "but"

F. Owners' Manual

Parents often state that they were not given an Owners' Manual when the child was born. We are providing you with a card that can be laminated and put in your wallet or purse to remind you of the choices you have in parenting your child. Each of the strategies in the Owners' Manual is reviewed in Chapters 2–5.

Table 3

OWNERS' MANUAL
INCREASE POSITIVES: ATTEND TO YOUR CHILD'S APPROPRIATE BEHAVIOR
FRONT LOAD YOUR CHILD: MAKE SURE YOUR CHILD UNDERSTANDS WHAT IS EXPECTED OF THEM BEFORE IMPLEMENTING A BEHAVIORAL STRATEGY
POST RULES AND USE PICTURES AS VISUAL REMINDERS
"YOU HAVE A DIRECTION TO__________."
GIVE AN EMPATHETIC STATEMENT
USE DAILY REPORT CARD
USE TOKEN SYSTEM
PACKAGING
MODEL APPROPRIATE BEHAVIOR
NO FREEBIES
USE TIME-OUT
TAKE AWAY A PRIVILEGE OR POINTS/RESONSE COST
IGNORE MINOR INAPPROPRIATE BEHAVIOR
PROMPT YOUR CHILD
MAKE A PLAN FOR PARENTING IN PUBLIC

Summary Parenting Steps

We are not parenting our children in a vacuum free from life's challenges. While the parenting strategies reviewed in the previous chapters seem easy, they become more complex with all our daily distractions. It is just as important to realize the potential missteps that can occur, as it is to learn the parenting strategies themselves. Only once we recognize when we have taken a misstep can we avoid unnecessary setbacks. Missteps are natural; it is how we manage to recognize and avoid them that will prevent us from becoming derailed.

A. Always Dance with the One You Came With: Divide and Conquer

It is hard for parents to always be on the same page on how to best parent their child. If you do not present a united front with your child, they will naturally look for the parent who will agree with them. All disagreements between parents should be done in private. Always check with your child to see if they have already gotten an answer to their question from the other parent.

B. Dancing with an Audience: Don't Change the Steps When Performing in Public

We all try to avoid embarrassing situations. We need to recognize that children are uninhibited and if left to their own devices will choose to do things that will embarrass us. As parents, we need to teach our children what is acceptable behavior in public and follow through with consequences even though others are watching. Children need to learn that the same rules that apply at home also apply in public.

C. Learning to Dance with Others: Out of Sight, Out of Mind

Parents control a wide range of powerful reinforcers that can be used to influence their child's behavior in settings outside of the home. A simple daily report card (DRC) can be used to get feedback from others who are supervising your child. A DRC can be a practical way of providing motivation for your child to comply with teachers, neighbors, and coaches. They provide you with feedback on how your child behaved through the DRC and you provide the consequences, both positive and negative, at home.

D. Good Days and Bad Days

We all have "good days" and "bad days." Our daily responsibilities can wear us down. This is not the time to evaluate how things are going with our children. Invariably we would say Terribly. Objectively, this may not be accurate but merely a reflection of how we are feeling. We all need to find a way to take time for ourselves and rejuvenate. When we feel good we may view life in a very different way.

E. A Special Case of the "Yeah, Buts"

When we hear ourselves saying, "I know I should have handled the situation differently, but…," we need to take our own advice and eliminate the "buts." Do what we know we should have done! Often we know what to do but let things get in the way of doing them.

CHAPTER 6

Helping Your Child Make Friends

Looking out the kitchen window I could see my seven-year-old son Jack watching two boys playing basketball in their driveway. He wants desperately to make friends. I envisioned him walking up to the two boys and asking if he could play next. He would joke with them and praise their good shots. When they finished their game they would ask Jack to play.

In reality it didn't go as I envisioned. I could see by the look on his face that he really wanted to join them. He slowly walked over to where the boys were playing and stood waiting for them to notice him. He didn't say anything and just stood there watching. I could see him becoming discouraged. He lowered his head and walked away. My poor boy looked dejected. I could feel his disappointment and wanted to do something to help him.

In fact, parents are in the best position to actually help their child by addressing real problems they observe on a daily basis. Jack's father envisioned how Jack could engage the boys playing basketball and join in their game. He could see what Jack needed to learn if he was going to be able to join into a future basketball game. Jack needs to learn to stand on the sideline and wait until he is acknowledged. He needs to learn to genuinely praise good shots.

Jack also needs to learn to ask if he can join the game and wait for an answer. If they say, "Not now," he needs to come back later and try again. Dad can role-play this scenario with Jack and prompt him to try again. He can set up a play-date with several boys to play one-on-one basketball so the boys have to take turns playing. His Dad can join the game and model what they role-played and reinforce Jack for his efforts in taking turns, praising good shots, and patiently waiting for his turn.

Helping Children Find Dance Partners

We have used dancing as a metaphor for parenting because it reflects the reciprocal relationship between parents and their children. Dancing can also serve as a metaphor for the interaction between children as they try to form friendships. Imagine if you went to a dance and no one wanted to dance with you. What if you were too shy to approach anyone at the dance? How might people respond to you if you were extremely aggressive and demanded that someone dance with you? What impression would people have of you if you asked someone to dance and they said, "No," but you kept nagging them to dance with you? In each of these scenarios we can feel the disappointment and sadness one would feel if his/her efforts to find a dance partner were rejected.

Parents as Choreographers: Strategies to Help Children Make Friends

Some children are better at making friends than others. All children have problems making and keeping friends at some time. Parents are in an excellent position to help their children gain social competence and meet the challenges of making friends. What better place to learn to interact with others than in the natural setting of the home, park, or playground? We can watch our children playing and can see when things don't go well. We can then structure future play-dates as opportunities to teach them new ways of responding to difficult situations and help them learn how to make friends. The observations we make can become the content of what we teach our children. We can then influence the behavioral choices our children make in playing with other children through the skills we learned in the preceding chapters.

There are many areas where children may need help in learning to make friends. Some children may not have sensitivity to the needs of others and are egocentric. They do not recognize how children are feeling and fail to read children's body language. Children may not have sufficient communication skills to communicate effectively with their peers. They become frustrated and angry because their peers do not seem to understand them. Some children may have an aggressive disposition and frighten other children. Children may be extremely sensitive to teasing and may become the target for bullies. Children may lack self-confidence and shy away from approaching children they would like to befriend. There are several strategies that parents can use to focus on teaching children how to connect with other children and form friendships.

Reading Body Language and Facial Expressions

Some children have difficulty reading others' body language and facial expressions. They are unaware of what another child may be feeling and charge ahead clueless to the fact that their behavior may be inappropriate given how the other child feels. If they were able to read the other child's body language, they may have approached the situation differently. For example, a child may have his/her arms crossed and a frown on his face. His/her body language says, "I'm angry. Stay away." If a child approaches him/her who does not read his/her body language, the child may be in danger of getting hit or pushed away. Children need to learn when it is best to approach another child, and when it is not.

The most effective way to teach children to read body language as well as other children's emotions is in the moment. Parents can take the opportunity to ask their child how they think someone is feeling based on how they appear. "Look at John's face. How do you think he is feeling?" "His face looks angry." "Susan has her head down. How do you think she is feeling?" "She looks sad." "Mark is smiling. How do you think he is feeling?" "He seems happy."

To help your child recognize how body language can tell you how a person might react, you can ask him/her to tell you what might happen if you approach the other child based on how the child looks. "Do you think John wants to play now?" "Would this be a good time to talk to John?" This is a first step in helping your child in understanding someone else's perspective.

Showing Interest in Someone Else

Parents can also teach their child how to ask questions of the other children to connect with them and understand their interests. "What games do you like to play?" "What is your favorite food?" "What are your favorite television shows?" "Do you play video games?" "What video games do you like to play?" This information can be used in planning a play-date. You can encourage him/her to try playing something that the other child said he/she liked. Have them notice how the other child responds when playing a favorite game. You can then reinforce him/her for considering the other child's preferences and playing a game they chose. Over time they will learn to consider the interest of their peers in a play-date.

Modeling Social Behavior

In Chapter 3, we learned the importance of modeling. Parents can have a mock play-date with their child, focusing on modeling the social behaviors that their child needs to learn. For example, if your child does not give eye contact and greet other children, you could model this for them. Before starting a play session, you can have your child give you eye contact and greet you using the greeting you modeled. Modeling is an efficient way of teaching everything at once. Your child can learn the appropriate tone of voice, demeanor in greeting someone, and what to say just by watching you model for him.

Self-as-a-Model

A second strategy is through the use of video. iPads, iPhones, and digital cameras can all be used to create videos as models of appropriate social behavior. A technique called self-as-a-model can increase the effectiveness of modeling. In self-as-a-model the parent videotapes his/her child successfully demonstrating the social behavior he/she wants him/her to learn. You can do this by modeling what you want him/her to do and videotaping him/her doing it. You can then edit the segment of the video showing him/her successfully demonstrating the behavior. Once you have a sample tape of him/her, you can use the tape as a model for him/her to view prior to a play-date. Self-as-a-model is effective because it eliminates the problems often associated with modeling. If your child sees someone else modeling the behavior, he/she can say, "Sure he/she can do it, but I can't." He/she may see the model as an expert and feel incapable of doing what the expert can do. With self-as-a-model, he/she can't say that because he/she is the model demonstrating the skill. This can be used for any social behavior you want to target. Another advantage is that children like seeing themselves on videotape.

Models through TV and Movies

Another strategy for teaching appropriate social behavior is through select television shows. Kids love to watch TV. Parents can sit with them and analyze the interactions of the actors in a movie or characters in a cartoon. The actors and characters demonstrate both positive and negative examples of how to handle various social situations. While sitting with your child, you can probe him/her with questions about how the actor or cartoon character could have handled the same situations better. You can also focus on good models of social behaviors.

Watching TV offers an opportunity to practice reading body language by helping your child recognize the clues that tell you how someone feels. If you are able to watch superheroes that your child admires, you can use them as a prompt during a play-date. For example, you might say, "How would Spider-Man handle this situation?"

Choreographing the Dance: Setting Up Play-Dates

The first step in helping your child develop skills in playing with others is observation. Setting up a play-date and observing what your child is doing that is negatively effecting his/her relationship with others can help you pinpoint what your child needs to do to be more successful. You may notice that your child lacks awareness and sensitivity of how his/her social behavior affects others. It may be that he/she has not learned the skills of socially engaging his/her peers. On the other hand, he/she may have the skills but not use them in the appropriate context. In this section we have provided a rating scale to help you identify potential problems and a planning sheet for setting up and structuring a play-date. After observing your child playing with other children several times, fill out the rating scale and prioritize the skills you will focus on teaching your child. Once you know what the problem is, you are in a position to structure a play-date to help your child learn new skills and begin to make friends. The more positive experiences your child has with another child, the more likely he will be able to foster a friendship.

Planning a Play-Date

Parents frequently arrange play-dates for their children. Sometimes the play-dates do not go well. If this is the case, planning ahead can avoid unnecessary problems. Instead of ending the play-date when someone is crying, fighting, or hurt, with planning, it can end on a positive note with the guest wanting to come back for another play-date. We have provided a rating scale identifying problems that children often have in playing with other children. By rating your child's behavior, you can identify potential problems using Table 1. Any items rated 5 or greater are problems that your child has in playing with other children. Using Table 2, you can create a successful play-date that addresses these problems.

Table 1

PROBLEM CHECKLIST FOR PLAY-DATE

PROBLEM CHECK LIST FOR PLAY-DATE										
Child's Name: Jack										
Rater: Alan										
	No Problem									Problem
	1	2	3	4	5	6	7	8	9	10
Is bossy with other children										
Tries to control the activity										
Is passive and controlled by others										
Does not choose to stay engaged with other children										
Is physically aggressive with other children (deliberately hurts others)										
Teases other children										
Brags to other children										
Quits game when things don't go their way										
Doesn't share with other children										
Doesn't like to take turns										
Focuses on winning										
Doesn't clean up after game										
Changes the rules of a game in order to win										

Doesn't follow the rules of a game or activity										
Doesn't cooperate with other children										
Likes to show off for other children										
Lies during a play activity										
Uses inappropriate language (cursing or swearing)										
Accidently hurts other children (clumsy or unaware)										
Cries when loses or gets out in a game or activity										
Hogs the ball or materials of an activity										
Excludes others from a game or activity										
Has difficulty joining in on a game or activity										
Wants their own way										
Isn't willing to problem-solve										
Cheats when playing a game or activity										
Doesn't listen to others in a conversation										
Dominates conversations										
Overly focused on one topic in a conversation										
Doesn't recognize someone is not interested in their topic of conversation										
Plays alone, leaving the other child by themselves										
Interrupts others' conversation										
Talks too loudly										
Defies adult direction										
Does not accept ending a play-date										

Does not transition back to parent when play-date ends										
LIST ALL ITEMS THAT ARE RATED A 5 OR GREATER:										

Table 2

PLANNING A SUCCESSFUL PLAY-DATE

Parent(s):

Play-date participants:

Play-date:

Length of playtime:

What activity/activities will they do?

How will you structure the environment?

How will you structure the activity?

What reinforcers can the children earn during the activity?

What are the rules of the activity?

What social skill will you focus on during the play-date?

What are the anticipated problems and your proposed solutions?

Problems:

Solutions:

Planning for the Play-Date

Once you have identified the problem behaviors that are causing your child to have difficulty playing with other children, you can plan the next play-date. Remember, the goal is to have the other child want to return for another play-date. Your child needs to be sensitive to the preferences of his/her guest so he/she can create a fun play-date.

Setting the Occasion for Success

The goal of planning a play-date is to practice preparing your child for an activity to increase the probability of their success. Often we develop a plan for an activity without making sure that our child fully understands it or has the skills to do it. Taking the time to brief your child will increase the probability that your child will have a successful play-date. The following table provides some suggested steps in preparing your child for an activity.

Steps for Preparing Your Child for a Play-Date

1. Pick a time when your child is relaxed and ready to communicate with you.

   Using "no freebies" can help to motivate your child to participate in planning a play-date. "First we're going to discuss your play-date with John and than you can go out and play."

   Time: ___________. Place: ___________________________.

2. Help your child develop a plan for playing with the visiting child. Make sure he/she understands that the goal of the play-date is to have a fun time, so that the visiting child will want to come back to play with him/her again. "What would the other child like to do?" "Can we come up with several ideas for activities that both of you might enjoy?" "What if your guest wants to do something different than you want to do, what could we do?" Including your child in the planning will help him/her learn to problem-solve and create a greater interest in the plan.

3. Review the play-date plan you developed together in a simple and concise manner. To make sure your child understands the plan, probe for understanding. "Can you tell me how you can earn extra TV time?" "How long is the play-date?" "What if you want to play a different game than your friend?" Make sure that you praise your child for attempting to answer your questions. You can also ask the questions in the form of a game. "I'm going to test you on what I just said and you can earn a penny for every correct answer."

4. If you are still not sure that your child understands the plan or whether he/she has the skill to implement the plan, you can role-play with him/her. For example, you could role-play accepting when another child wants to play a different game than your child. "Let's pretend I am Josh and you ask me if I want to play Uno. I say, 'No, I want to play checkers'. Show me what you would say and do." Make sure the role-play situation is exactly what your child will be doing during the play-date.

Do the role-play in the setting where the children will be playing and use the same materials that will be available to them.

5. Ask your child if they have any questions about the plan. If they have suggestions that you can incorporate, then add them to the plan for the play-date. If your child comes up with ways to handle situations, they will have more buy-in to the plan.

Putting It All Together: Dad Choreographs a Play-Date for Jack with Mark

Alan is Jack's Dad. He has been watching Jack from a distance and is concerned about Jack. He knows Jack wants to have friends but doesn't know how to go about it. It is no wonder that he has no friends the way he treats his peers. Alan decides to take steps to teach Jack how to make friends.

Since he watched Jack recently with Mark, he has an idea of the problems. He also decides to use a rating scale, Table 1, the Problem Checklist for Playdate above, to make sure he identifies the most serious problems:

The following items from table 1 were rated 5 or above:

1. Tries to control the activity
2. Does not choose to stay engaged with other children
3. Quits game when things don't go their way
4. Doesn't share with other children
5. Doesn't cooperate with other children
6. Hogs the ball or materials of an activity
7. Doesn't like to take turns
8. Excludes others from a game or activity
9. Has difficulty joining in on a game or activity
10. Wants their own way
11. Doesn't listen to others in a conversation
12. Dominates conversations

13. Doesn't recognize someone is not interested in their topic of conversation
14. Plays alone, leaving the other child by themselves
15. Interrupts others' conversation

Alan decides to target the following social behaviors based on his observations and the rating scale:

1. Greeting the guest at the door.
2. Giving undivided attention to the guest.
3. Asking questions about what the guest likes and listening to his/her answers.
4. Being willing to do what the guest wants to do.
5. Making genuinely supportive positive comments to the guest.
6. Taking turns in a game.

Next, Alan decides to fill out the Planning a Successful Play-Date form to develop a plan for helping Jack.

PLANNING A SUCCESSFUL PLAY-DATE

Parent(s): Alan

Play-date participants: Jack and Mark

Play-date: 8-3-2014

Length of playtime?

One hour

What activity/activities will they do?
They will select from several things that Mark states he would like to do. If Mark has trouble thinking of things to do, Jack will offer

playing computer games, playing pool, riding bikes, or watching a video together.

How will you structure the environment?
If Mark and Jack decide to ride bikes I will tell them where they can ride. They need to wear bike helmets and let me know where they will ride. If Mark chooses computer games, Jack will select several computer games for Mark to choose from.

How will you structure the activity?
Jack will greet Mark and invite him into the house. He will ask Mark to come into the living room so they can talk about what they want to do. Jack will suggest several possible activities: computer games, pool, bike riding, or watching a movie. He will listen to Mark and repeat back what Mark says. If Mark has another idea that they could do, Jack will accept Mark's idea. Jack will make positive comments about Mark in the activity.

What reinforcers can the children ean during the activity?
I will use a report card to give Jack feedback on his social behaviors during the chosen activity. I will ask Jack to meet with me briefly to go over his report card every twenty minutes. The feedback should take no more than ten to twenty seconds. He will get feedback on how well he is doing during that twenty-minute period on the following behaviors:

1. Greeting the guest at the door.
2. Giving undivided attention to the guest.
3. Asking questions about what the guest likes and listening to his answers.
4. Being willing to do what the guest wants to do.
5. Making genuinely supportive positive comments to the guest.
6. Taking turns in a game.

He will earn 1–5 points on each item. Five means he did the behavior 100 percent of the time when appropriate. One means he did the behavior 10 percent of the time or less when appropriate.

He will earn 0–5 pts. for greeting Mark at the door since there is only one opportunity to greet Mark. Since Jack expressed that he wanted to stay up later as a reward, he will have an opportunity to earn extra bedtime based on the points he earns on the report card.

Important note: The chart needs to be made child friendly. Children will be more likely to show interest in the chart if they are involved in creating it. Three strategies that can increase children's interest in the chart are:

1. Have your child draw a picture of them-selves completing each task for use in the chart.
2. Take pictures of them completing each task for use in the chart.
3. Have them decorate the chart.

Greet guest at the door	5			
Undivided attention to guest	1 2 3 4 5	1 2 3 4 5	1 2 3 4 5	1 2 3 4 5
Asking questions of guest and listening	1 2 3 4 5	1 2 3 4 5	1 2 3 4 5	1 2 3 4 5
Supportive comments	1 2 3 4 5	1 2 3 4 5	1 2 3 4 5	1 2 3 4 5
Taking turns and doing what the quest chooses	1 2 3 4 5	1 2 3 4 5	1 2 3 4 5	1 2 3 4 5
			Total Points	
Reward	80–70 One hour extra bedtime	69–59 Half hour extra bedtime	58–48 Fifteen minutes extra bedtime	47 and below Regular bedtime

What are the rules of the activity?

1. Mark is the guest at our house and he gets to choose the activity they will do.
2. Jack will stay with the activity once they agree on what they will do.
3. Jack will make an effort to make Mark feel welcome by making positive comments to Mark during the play-date.
4. During a game or activity Mark will take turns and share materials.
5. Jack will listen to Mark and question Mark if he does not understand something that Mark has said.

What social skill will you focus on during the play-date?

1. Greeting a guest
2. Playing a game that a guest chooses.
3. Listening to a guest.
4. Taking turns in a game.
5. Staying with the game.
6. Making positive supportive statements to a guest.

What are the anticipated problems and your proposed solutions?

Problems:

1. Jack will not greet his guest or will greet his guest without enthusiasm.
2. Jack will not want to play what his guest chooses and choose what he wants to do.
3. Jack will leave his guest and play alone if his guest chooses something he does not want to play.
4. Jack will not listen to or say anything positive to his guest.
5. Jack will dominate play and not take turns during a game.

Solutions: Through the use of a report card system, Jack will earn points for appropriate social behaviors. He will get quick feedback on how he is doing at twenty-minute intervals as a motivation to earn all the points possible on his report card. I will also role-play the targeted appropriate social behaviors several times during the week prior to Mark coming over. I will use video clips for Jack to look at prior to each of our role-plays and Mark coming over to play as an additional prompt for Jack.

Preparing Jack for the Play-Date

Now that Alan has a plan he decides to practice with Jack. He tells Jack, "We're going to practice having Mark come over for a play-date." Jack is playing with his video and ignores Dad. Dad says, "You have a direction to give me your iPad in ten minutes." "You need to stop in ten minutes." Jack doesn't appear to have heard Dad. Dad says, "What did I say?" Jack answers, "I have to give you the iPad in ten minutes." Dad gives him several quick reminders as the time winds down. Jack hands Dad the iPad. Alan says, "I know it's hard to stop playing a game on the iPad, but you did great stopping. We are going to plan together for your play-date with Mark. When we're done planning, we are going to go over the plan and role-play."

Dad decided not to criticize Jack's poor social behavior at his last play-date but to focus on how to make it better. He did not want to make Jack feel bad. Jack needs to learn better social behavior in playing with peers. He is not aware of how his behavior affects his peers.

Dad started with the importance of greeting your guest. He told Jack that it was important to give your guest eye contact, smile and welcome him to the house. Next, Dad role-played with Jack pretending to be Jack. Jack was asked to pretend he was Mark and to knock on the door and wait for Dad to greet him. Jack went outside, knocked on the door and Dad opened the door, looked Jack in the eyes, smiled and said, "Come on in." He then asked Jack how his greeting made him feel? Jack said, "Good." Dad then asked Jack to pretend he was Mark, and he wanted Jack to greet him just as he was greeted. Dad, pretending to be Mark, knocked on the door and Jack opened the door. Jack looked at Dad and unenthusiastically said, "Come in." Dad said, "Let's do this again, but this time smile and say it like you mean it." Dad once again knocked on the door. Jack opened the door, looked at Dad, smiled and said, "Come in." Dad said, "That's great! Let's video-tape this." Jack perked up and said, "Really?" Dad said, "Sure, that was a great role-play and I want to tape it." They repeated the scene and Dad taped it.

Next, Dad said, "Let's think of games or things Mark would like to do. Jack, how can you find out what Mark wants to do?" "I can ask him." "Okay, let's pretend I'm Mark and you can ask me what I want to do. Let me try it first, I'll pretend to be you and you be Mark." Dad said, "Let's talk in the living room." Dad looked Jack in the eyes and asked, "Mark, what's your favorite thing to do?" Jack said, "I like to play computer games?" Dad said, "Oh, you like computer games." Jack said "Yeah." Dad said, "Would you like to see my games? We could take turns playing a game." Dad stopped the role-play and asked, "How did you feel when I asked you what you wanted to play?" "I really liked it." Dad said, "That's right, you were a guest and I wanted you to have fun, so I agreed to play computers." "I also repeated what you said to make sure I understood what you wanted to do and you knew I was listening to you. Now you try it." Jack looked Dad in the eye and asked him to follow him to the living room where they could talk. Jack said, "Mark, what do you like to do?" Dad said, "I like to play basketball." Jack said, "No, we're going to play computer games." Dad stopped the role-play. "You were doing good until I said I wanted to play basketball. You said, 'No, let's play computers.' Remember, you invited Mark over to play with you, you need to make it fun. You may need to play basketball if you want Mark to choose to come over for a play-date in the future. You could say, 'Is it okay if we play basketball for awhile and then we can play computers?' Let's try it again." Jack asked Dad pretending to be Mark to follow him to the living room and they could decide what they wanted to play. Jack asked Dad, "What do want to play?" Dad said, "Basketball." Jack said, "Okay, after we play basketball can we play computer games?" Dad said, "Sure." "That was great, let's videotape the role-play." Jack agreed and they videotaped the role-play. They also role-played playing basketball and videotaped examples of Jack praising Dad when he made good shots.

Report Card: How Am I Doing?

"One more thing we are going to practice, a report card for the play-date." Jack looked surprised, "What do you mean a report card?" Dad explained that he was going to give Jack feedback on whether he remembered what they role-played. Every twenty minutes Dad was going to ask Jack to privately meet with him briefly to rate how Jack was doing in his play-date. Before Jack could protest, Dad said if he did well on his report card he could earn a later bedtime. Jack's eyes widened with enthusiasm and he said, "Really?" Dad said, "Sure, if you try hard with the things we worked on, you deserve to stay up later. You can earn up to one hour added to your normal bedtime." He then showed Jack the report card and explained how it worked. Next, Dad role-played with Jack, marking the report card.

Preparing for the Play-Date

Dad role-played the components of the play-date and reviewed the video clips several times during the week. He answered all questions Jack had about the play-date and report card. They also watched several TV programs together and practiced trying to read the body language of the actors and commenting on things the actors did well or could have done better.

The Play-Date

Jack earned thirty minutes of extended time before bedtime. The preparations greatly improved the quality of Jack's play-date, and Mark agreed to another play-date. Dad and Jack reviewed what went well and what Jack could have done better. They agreed on creating several additional role-plays and videos to practice for the next play-date. Jack was excited to have another play-date with Mark.

Concluding Thoughts on Play-Dates

Parents are in the best position to observe and help their children improve their social behavior. Helping your child learn how to make friends and get along with others will help them throughout their lives, at home, school, and eventually in the workplace. The earlier you start, the better. With the skills you learned in the previous chapters and this chapter, you no longer have to stand by helplessly watching your child wishing he/she had friends. You can take an active role in choreographing his/her success.

Planning a Birthday Party

Birthday parties are celebrated with friends. By planning ahead, birthday parties can be fun and something to look forward to. A well-planned birthday party can help your child strengthen his/her friendships. The following is a planning form that can help prevent catastrophe.

Planning a Birthday Party

How many kids will I invite?

What should the ratio of adult supervision to child be?

What activities will I have?

Are there children who are too young or too old for the activity? (If yes) What will they do?

How can I schedule the party to reduce downtime?

What rules do I need to control the activities and address potential problems?

Who gets to open the presents?

What if my child does not like his presents or gets more than one of the same presents?

Do I need rules for the games we play to ensure safety?

How do I handle aggressive behavior?

Will I require the parents to attend the party?

Is there anything that might hurt someone or get ruined or broken that I need to remove?

What if my child wants to exclude certain children? Do I invite everyone from his school or only certain children?

Who will be in charge of the various activities: games, food, opening gifts, etc.?

Are there areas of the house or grounds that are off limits?

How will I control transitions from one activity to another?

Teaching Children Skills to Get Along with Others

In the previous sections we presented strategies for helping your child make friends through structured play-dates. Children also need skills to support their general interactions with other children and adults. The University of California at Irvine (UCI), Child Development Center (CDC) has developed a social skills curriculum to help children get along with others. Children learn to be assertive as opposed to aggressive or passive in asking for things. They learn how to be good sports in games. They learn that sometimes it is better to accept a situation than to fight it and that accepting is a proactive choice. They learn how to ignore provocation. Finally, they learn how to problem-solve so they can help themselves in difficult situations.

Children who learn to use these skills are better prepared to get along with others. The UCI-CDC has also developed a set of strategies designed to help parents teach these skills in daily situations. First, we will define each of the skills and then learn strategies to teach them.

Styles of Communication

Children often request things of their parents, teachers, and peers. How they ask can increase the probability that they will get what they want or at least be heard. There are three possible styles children might use in asking for something: assertive, aggressive, or passive. The first goal in teaching your child to be assertive is to make sure they know the difference between these styles of interaction. We never want them to model aggressive or passive styles of communication but we do want them to recognize the difference. Sometimes a child might think they are being assertive when in fact they are being aggressive or passive. Their style of communication is not a choice if they do not know the difference. In order to discern the different styles of communication, the child first learns how someone would appear if they were using each style. What would they be saying? What would their demeanor look like? How close would they be standing to the person they are talking to? Where would they be looking? How loud would they be speaking? The answers to these questions would tell you the style they are using.

Assertive Style Characteristics

An assertive person's communication would be direct and clear. He/she would speak in a normal tone of voice. He/she would have a calm body. He/she would look the person in the eyes when speaking to them. He/she would a have a relaxed face and smile. He/she would also respect the individual's personal space. Imagine a bubble around the person at least an arm's length away from them. He/she would not cross into their bubble.

Aggressive Style Characteristics

An aggressive communication would sound harsh or angry. The person would speak in a loud tone of voice. He/she would be demanding and appear to glare at the person. He/she would be stiff and tense. He/she would not respect the individual's personal space.

Passive Style Characteristics

A passive communication would be unclear, unintelligible, and tentative. The person would speak in a soft, low tone of voice. He/she would not give the person he/she is talking to eye contact. He/she would have his/her head down and appear nervous. He/she would be standing at a more-than-necessary distance from the person he/she is talking to.

Teaching Children to Know the Difference

One strategy is to use puppets. Puppets are given names that represent each style. "Cool Craig" is the assertive puppet. "Mean Max" is the aggressive puppet. "Wimpy Wally" is the passive puppet. Using puppets increases children's willingness to participate in the training. Even more important, once the children learn to identify the styles of communication with the name of the puppets, you can quickly cue them to change their style of communication. For example, if you see your child being a "Mean Max," you can quickly prompt him to change his/her behavior by saying, "Remember to be a Cool Craig." You don't have to go over all the individual characteristics of each style. The use of the puppet's name brings a complete picture of the style represented by the puppet.

You can teach children to distinguish the communication styles by modeling each style with the puppets and asking them whether the puppet was a "Cool Craig," "Mean Max," or "Wimpy Wally." Ask them to tell you which style of communication the puppet was using and why. Once they have learned to recognize the styles using the puppets, you can have them model being a "Cool Craig." Remember, you do not want them to practice being a "Mean Max," or "Wimpy Wally." You can also choose select TV programs to watch and identify the different styles of communication.

Good Sportsmanship

The first step in teaching your child to be a good sport is to identify the characteristics of someone who is a good sport. A good sport is someone who uses a "Cool Craig" voice. They ask others to join in the game when they ask to play. They follow the rules of a game. They accept when they are out in a game. They take turns in a game and share materials with others. They make encouraging statements to others. They help others if they are having trouble learning the game.

Teaching Good Sportsmanship

Parents can focus on good sportsmanship by playing games with their children and rating the game. A "Good Sports Thermometer" can be used after each game to rate the game, on a scale of 1–5. A 1 means that the person was not a good sport most of the time and a 5 means they were a good sport all of the time. Before rating the overall game, the parent and child rate the individual skills to see if they match on the rating scale. If they do not match, they discuss their different views of how the game went. Parents can create a portable chart with each individual skill and the overall skill listed on the chart.

Important note: The chart needs to be made child friendly. Children will be more likely to show interest in the chart if they are involved in creating it. Three strategies that can increase children's interest in the chart are:

1. Have your child draw a picture of themselves completing each task for use in the chart.
2. Take pictures of them completing each task for use in the chart.
3. Have them decorate the chart.

Good Sport Thermometer

Cool Craig	1 2 3 4 5 N/A
Lets Others Play	1 2 3 4 5 N/A
Follows Rules of the Game	1 2 3 4 5 N/A
Accepts When They are Out	1 2 3 4 5 N/A
Takes Turns in a Game	1 2 3 4 5 N/A
Shares Materials	1 2 3 4 5 N/A
Makes Encouraging Statements to Others	1 2 3 4 5 N/A
Helps Others in the Game	1 2 3 4 5 N/A
Good Sport	1 2 3 4 5

One strategy to motivate children to try to be good sports is the use of a "Good Sport Pizza Chart." The chart is a pizza with a designated number of pepperonis drawn on it. If the child earns a 4 on the Good Sport Thermometer he gets one pepperoni. If he earns a 5 he gets 2 pepperonis. As soon as all the pepperonis are colored in, the family has a pizza party to celebrate.

This strategy can also be included during a play-date. You can prompt your child that he/she can earn a pepperoni on the pizza if he/she is a good sport during the play-date. You can meet with him/her at the end of the play-date and rate his/her good sportsmanship on the Good Sport Thermometer. During the play-date you can use a simple hand sign to evaluate how the game is going. Every fifteen minutes you can give a thumbs up if your child has earned a 5 during that period, a thumb to the side if they are earning a 3, or thumbs down if they are earning less than a 3. The rating can serve to prompt your child to improve his/her behavior or reinforce him/her for being a good sport. This is a portable system that can be used in a variety of situations.

Accepting

This is a skill that is not often taught to children. Children think that things happen to them and they do not have a choice in how to react. One proactive choice is to accept. Sometimes your parents direct you to do something and they expect you to do it. One choice is to say "no," and to refuse to comply with them. Another choice is to accept their direction and do what they ask. What will happen to you if you refuse to comply with them? What will happen if you comply and accept the direction? Which is a better choice? Once children realize that they have a choice in how they respond, they are more likely to make a positive choice for themselves.

Children are taught exactly what they would be doing and saying if they were accepting. They would do what their parent directed them to do without complaining. They would be a "Cool Craig."

Ignoring Provocation

Children are often the targets of teasing. They are easily provoked. Bullies like to tease other children who respond to their taunting. If a child who is being teased does not respond in any way, it is likely that the bully will stop. The bully also may escalate their behavior, bringing attention to themselves, and may get in trouble. Children need to practice the art of ignoring, since it is not as easy as it sounds. Any reaction from the person being teased can encourage further teasing. Parents can role-play situations in which their child is being teased. After the role-play the parent and child can rate their performance on a 1–5 scale as to how they did in ignoring the teasing. A 1 means the child did not ignore the teaser. A 5 means they totally ignored the teaser. The parent and child can also rate the role-play and see if they match. If they do not match they can discuss why they disagree.

Problem-Solving

Once children learn the skills of assertion, accepting, good sportsmanship, and ignoring provocation, they are ready to learn to problem-solve. Parents can teach them several steps in problem-solving. The first step is to state the problem. What is causing a problem for them? Next, what are three possible solutions? Choose one. After the child tries their choice, evaluate whether it worked or not. To help children practice problem-solving, teach them to give you a sign when they have a problem and want to problem-solve. They can make a "T" with their hands to say, "I want to problem-solve." When you see them give you the sign, have them walk over to you and go through the problem-solving steps in private. For example, if your child is playing a game and another child won't let him have a turn, he might give you the problem-solving sign. If he can't remember the steps, help him to remember. The significant step is that he did not act impulsively and chose to problem-solve before acting. Ask him, "What is the problem?" "Johnny won't let me have a turn." "What are three possible solutions?" "I can accept. I can ask him in a Cool Craig way if I can have a turn. I can walk away and ignore him." "What do you choose?" "I am going to ask him in a Cool Craig way if I can play." " What is your second choice if that doesn't work?" "I am going to ignore him." "Okay, go try your choice and let me know if it works." Giving the problem-solving sign stops the action before the problem escalates and helps the child think of the best way to solve his/her problem. The parent does not solve the problem, the child comes up with choices he has been taught to solve his own problem.

Big Deal Fiesta

A practical token system that can be used throughout the day to focus on reinforcing your child for using any of the social skills they have learned is a Big Deal chart. Big Deals are simply points in the form of stickers. Each time you see your child using one of the skills, you can tell him/her he/she earned a Big Deal towards a Big Deal Fiesta. When they earn enough Big Deals the family will have a fiesta with games and a special meal to celebrate how well the child is doing. In order to give you flexibility in when they can earn the Fiesta, you tell them that it is a magic number of Big Deals. You can start by giving them a Big Deal Fiesta when you think it would be optimal. For example, after an especially good day of earning Big Deals, you could decide to announce that they have earned a Big Deal Fiesta. This could hook them on earning Big Deals. On the average, after the first two Fiestas, children should earn them once a month. The Big Deals are portable and can be given any time you see them using their skills.

Taking an Active Role in Helping Your Child Make Friends and Get Along With Others

Parents want to see their child make friends and get along with other people. We can stand on the sidelines and hope that our child somehow develops the skills that will help him/her accomplish this goal, or we can take an active part in teaching him/her the skills. This chapter presented techniques that parents can use to help their child make friends with other children through structured play-dates. A format for planning successful birthday parties was also presented. Parents can plan birthday parties to increase the probability that guests at the party will have a good time. A successful birthday party can help your child enjoy his/her friends and celebrate their friendship. Last, a format was presented for parents to use in teaching their child a set of social skills that can help them meet the social challenges of getting along with others. Taking the role of teacher is not easy, but can be extremely rewarding. You are in the best position to help your child meet the daily challenges life brings their way. Armed with the skills provided in this section, you no longer need to stand on the sideline. You can take an active role in helping your child make friends and get along with others.

SECTION III

CHAPTER 7

Transitions in the Dance Steps: Tweaking for the Pre-Teen and Teen Years

"As a parent, I possess tremendous power to make a child's life miserable or joyous. I can be a tool of torture or an instrument of inspiration. I can humiliate or humor, hurt or heal. In all situations it is my response that decides whether a crisis will be escalated or de-escalated, and a child humanized or dehumanized."
(p. 13)
Adapted quote of Haim Ginott

Introduction

That we have the ability and the power to escalate or de-escalate situations is a formidable thought to appreciate; it is a thought that as a parent one often considers, especially during the era of adolescence. This opening quotation (written by Haim Ginott, a respected psychologist and writer) was written initially for teachers, but we respectfully adjusted it to encompass parents as well. As parents, we all retain the ability (in most cases) to diffuse incidents and interact with our offspring in a positive and dignified manner. The following words could act as a guiding medium to all of us as we help our children navigate through the challenging ups and downs of adolescence.

"I miss those years. Our house was always a bastion of activity. Every evening, especially the weekends we had kids over. Either they were playing some sport on our driveway, playing billiards or Ping-Pong in the garage or just hanging out. They were a true joy to have around. That is not to say there were not any hard moments, but collectively, they were great days. Silence was definitely something we didn't experience during the teen years, but the activity was wonderful to live."

The teen years are often described by many as something to the effect of a human roller coaster ride (on steroids), likely causing any amusement aficionado to swoon in awe. Adolescence can truly be both the best and worst of times, a confusing and paradoxical state to be in. Some moments may feel as if one is walking on cloud nine while others may feel as though you're walking in the gutter. Amidst all of the twists and turns, one thing remains certain: this era will never be uneventful. Being successful during these years for both parent and child has a lot to do with how you and your teen learn to co-exist with one another. To be effective as parents, we must exercise a great deal of patience and skilled guidance while recognizing the special qualities and gifts that our teen brings to our lives. Ironically, although we all had to painstakingly traipse through this circus, we often forget what it was like. We sometimes even find ourselves responding in ways that closely parallel our parents' practices. We were likely angry at the choices they imposed upon us when we were younger, but surprisingly may find ourselves applying the same parenting strategies used on us years ago.

Parents often question why their loving child morphs into a very complicated teenager. Parents recognize and realize the developmental changes that are expected in their teen, but nonetheless struggle with accepting and dealing with the transformation. We now may be living with a young person who is more combative, critical of himself/herself and others (including his/her parents), and who seems far more imbalanced than he/she was in years past. Our teens may respond to their new life situations with much more trial and error than in their younger years, as they develop their identity and spread their wings of independence. As parents, we need to acknowledge and accept that our children will have to start making their own choices, some of which may not necessarily be the best. The changes we are witnessing are just normal outcomes of this time period. Parents should remind themselves not to take these changes personally, but respond in the best manner possible. Logically, it means that we need to grow up with our teens and in fact, make changes of our own. The relationships between parent and teen are reciprocal; both parties exert influence and are influenced by each other. Strong relationships require a give and take among all parties.

Teens do not automatically become spoiled and out of control, as some assume when they witness the onset of adolescence. While most parents are aware that adolescence is inevitably accompanied by changes in behavior sometimes, they are not prepared to adjust their parenting style. Nevertheless, changes in behavior don't just occur overnight. It is commonly accepted that if teens were not provided with structure, consistency, and the proper discipline needed when they were younger, the transition into their teen years may be an even harder adjustment. This is why it really is so important that as parents we establish rules, structure, and appropriate consequences for our children from a very early age. All of the previously highlighted ideas should give parents a stronger platform and foundation to help their child grow into a well-balanced adult.

The teen years bring to our families youth who are yearning for more independence. Some teens enter this era with the turbulence of a harsh winter storm. Their unpredictable and volatile behaviors challenge their parents who are not used to this seemingly unstable conduct. Most contemporary authors who study teen/parent relationships ascertain that as teens progress through adolescence and begin developing their identities, the parenting modality the parents employed will be challenged (behaviors, rewards, parenting beliefs and ideas, etc.). Teens need a little more space in which to grow and develop their new identity than they did when they were younger. This doesn't imply that the modalities we suggested in the past few chapters are irrelevant, but the approach will need to be tweaked so that the ideas will be more applicable for this age group. One way of viewing this predicament is the recognition that when we parent our teen we have to look at both sides of the coin. On the one hand, we have a wealth of behavioral strategies, which can be helpful in any situation. The strategies that we used in the past continue to have tremendous potency, especially when coupled with realistic expectations and collaboration. On the flip side of the coin, we must learn to understand what is developmentally appropriate for this age group, so we are able to interact most effectively. When we combine both sets of insights from the coin, we should produce a synergistic outcome.

For a moment let's be a fly on the wall inside of a typical household in the middle of an altercation. Mom is frustrated with her daughter because she hasn't completed her chores. Adding salt to the wound, her daughter is giving her a bit of attitude. *"You're grounded for life! I have had it with your smart-alecky, disrespectful attitude. You don't tell me what goes on in this house. You need to shape up!"* Although these are definitely not the most encouraging words that one would like to hear between a parent and her teen, they represent the kind of words that may be shared between most parents and teens in difficult times (sometimes the words can be even more hurtful). The teen years can be some of the most challenging years that we have with our offspring; however, they also can be some of the most rewarding. Chaos and frustration in the home, especially with teenagers, truly can be kept at bay when all know the expectations and the applicable but reasonable rules to follow. When parameters are clearly and reasonably established, and we do not become overreactive, most teens will settle in a bit more easily. Furthermore, when we allow our teens to be engaged in some of the rule-setting that we establish, it makes them more willing to follow through.

The mixture often requires an astute ability to communicate with our teens to help them take ownership and problem-solve their issues. During this time of transition teens are trying cognitively to reframe their world and their identities. This typically requires separating their identities from those of their parents. Parenting requires us to let go of some of our past ways and add to our arsenal of skills such as covert monitoring, perfecting communication/problem-solving, and becoming a proficient and realistic negotiator. We will discuss each of these areas further within this chapter.

Years ago, a parent was talking to both of us about her experiences with her teenage daughter. She was aggravated and feeling very incompetent and unloved. As she was talking, she eventually looked at both of us and remarked, "Do you know why God makes the teen years?" Both of us looked at her intently, anticipating a deep, Zen-like response. Instead, what we heard was not particularly Zen-like but rather humorously jaded. She chuckled and simply responded, "It is because our teens give us so much aggravation during those years that as parents, we are ready for them to leave the nest." We both smiled at her answer and then engaged in a conversation regarding why so many people feel it is harder to parent teens than any other age group. It is rather ironic that younger children view their parents as their heroes and caring role models, whereas teens often view their parents as overly intrusive and not to be trusted—a much more combative posture. In our view, it isn't necessarily harder, just different.

Adolescence 101: Becoming a Social Spy to Learn about Adolescence

Parental Control/Limits

Before discussing some specific parenting options for teens, it might be helpful to provide a basic overview of what some of the expected changes are that you will witness during this era. The dance may become livelier for the next several years, but you will have a clearer understanding of developmental changes that will follow. Although the following topics are not completely inclusive of what to expect during adolescence, we have selected several of the major transitional topics that are most relevant.

As parents, we need to realize that there are many (often undesirable) behaviors that our teens will exhibit, which are normal and to be expected during their development into adulthood. It should be expected that teens will begin distancing themselves from their parents and become more peer-focused. Friends will become the most important thing in their lives. That doesn't mean that your teen doesn't love you any more, but that there is a change in his/her focus. Most teens become a bit more self-conscious, and they will begin to respond to things differently. As we enter this period with our teens, we should try to avoid making several cardinal mistakes in our interactions. Some of these tenets include avoiding nagging whenever possible, steering clear of meaningless arguments, and avoiding excessive lecturing. All of these options typically produce ineffective results. We need to stay composed and focused on the issues on hand.

Parental control and limit setting

The issue of parental control and limit setting for adolescents is probably the largest concern that many parents experience. Parents seem to be very concerned about how and when to set limits on their teens. They also seem to be worried about what kind of limits to set and how they can evaluate and determine what limits their teen needs. Discussions with hundreds of parents reveal parental concerns regarding circumstances under which limits can or should be changed. Most parents want to try to display a consistent front, but also realize that some things need to be altered.

Discipline alternatives

Parents are also concerned about what form of discipline is most effective when adolescents do not abide by these limits. Most seem to be interested in learning new ways to respond to adolescents when they make poor choices in their lives. Many parents may recognize that a response to the poor choice of a younger child may not be as effective or appropriate with their teen. As noted earlier, most parents realize that they may need to re-think their parenting approach when their child enters this new era.

Wired for flight feathers

Of vital importance to understanding the parent/teen power struggle is the biological underpinning of the transition from child to teen. At this stage in their lives, adolescents are experiencing physical, cognitive, and emotional changes often simultaneously. As stated by Wolfe (1991):

"This turn toward independence, toward a world separate from family and home, has always been at the core of adolescence, today and a thousand years ago. It is an inevitable process. More than anything else, it is responsible for most of the behavior that constitutes adolescence."

As inevitable as these changes are, allowing a child to separate from you and create his/her own life can be very difficult for some parents. However, as a parent of a teenager, you really must develop an acceptance that allows your teen to make this necessary step. Traditionally, the first noticeable behavioral change that is witnessed is the teen beginning to argue more frequently. During this transition from childhood to adolescence, teens experience rapid cognitive growth. This enhanced capacity for reasoning manifests itself into seemingly constant arguing and questioning of the ideas and assumptions of parents that previously would not have started a quarrel. This can be confusing, infuriating, and hurtful to parents who are taken aback by the constant cross-examination and disagreements from their teen (APA, 2002). Developmental psychologists believe that this argumentative turn is actually quite healthy. The teens seem to use "their argumentativeness to work out their own values and their identity. In this way, the values and identity they eventually settle on feel like *theirs*, not someone else's" (Nowinski, 2007). The need for independence and finding their wings, as well as not following what they are told to do, is developmentally expected. Even if your teen eventually settles on the values that you have long espoused, this battling cognitive exercise to reach a decision is very important for a teen to learn. As Londergan (2008) succinctly writes:

"Newsflash: Not only do teens not have to like you, they're not even supposed to like you. Right now, it's our teens' job to snap the strong cords that still bind them to us so they can grow up and move away."

The importance of peers

Peer relationships become increasingly important. This change is often painful to parents who were used to being the ones from whom their children seek approval. This transition in support systems is to be expected, quite valuable, and very positive for teens. They greatly benefit from learning from each other. Just as teens can model negative behaviors from each other, they can also encourage positive behaviors and values (Moore & Zaff, 2002).

While the challenges and attempts to separate from you may be discouraging, parents should also remember that despite the explicit and implicit messages your teen may be sending you, your relationship with him/her is still crucial. Parents must strive to keep open lines of communication with their teens while continuing to communicate important information and values. Teens still need us to model behaviors for them as they enter this new territory that leads to adulthood. Although they really don't ask for it, they truly still need us to be mindful of what they are doing and help guide them with some basic rules and limits. Research shows that the teens brought up by parents who attend to these key points and maintain warm and caring relationships are more likely to be more adjusted psychologically and perform better educationally during this time of transition. (Moore & Zaff, 2002).

The search for identity

As expected, teenage identity is also an overarching concern for teens. Forming a new identity not only encompasses new emerging behaviors, thoughts, attire, and friends, but also presents a new way to interact with their families. These changes frustrate parents as they learn to adjust their level of involvement in their child's life (who is now growing up). As teens try to establish their identity, they will often seek the approval and counsel of their increasingly important and influential peer group. While parents may not always understand or agree with certain things that their teen will choose to engage in, we must reassure our teens that they have our support (of course, an adult perspective is always needed to ensure that the choices they make are safe and reasonable). The process of searching for a new identity is also known as individuation. Individuation occurs when teens join a group of peers that they seem to identify with closely, while at the same time becoming increasingly detached from and avoiding their interactions with their parents. As Nowinski (2007) advises:

"You can guide your children towards a healthy identity by accepting their current sense of who they are and, when opportunities arise, simply letting them know that they have choices, but don't try to steer them in a particular direction, or they may very well head the other way!"

This adolescent transformation of himself/herself can be affirming, amusing, or quite alarming for a parent. The changes in teens' behaviors and new identities can leave some of us doubting our teens' choices and wanting to tell him/her what to do. But teens seem biologically predisposed to try new things out, and unfortunately make some questionable decisions. Hopefully, they are safe decisions. They will receive comfort, however, from our continued love and support (Londergan, 2008). That is not to say that we will agree with all their choices and be happy with all the directions they choose to follow. Our job will be to continue to direct, but perhaps in a new manner. As Sachs states, "The elemental irony and mystery of child-rearing is that children are most likely to grow and change for the better only when they can trust that they'll be loved even if they stay the same."

Teenage drinking and substance abuse

According to the National Institute for Alcohol Abuse and Alcoholism (2013), by the age of fifteen more than half of teens have had at least one drink. By age eighteen the percentage of teens that have had at least one drink rises to 70 percent. Clearly, teenage drinking is a serious problem. Underage drinking is not only illegal but also harmful to the still-developing teenage brain; such harm can result in many future negative repercussions. Also, according to the Office of Adolescent Health of the US Dept. of Health & Human Services, by their senior year in high school, approximately half of adolescents have used an illicit drug at least once. Yes, these are rather frightening statistics but does this mean we should hunker down with our adolescents in our parenting survival bunkers until the storms of the teen years pass? Of course not. Not every adolescent will drink or experiment with drugs, and there still will be a percentage of teens that will abstain from both. However, the statistics clearly show how unrealistic it is to bury your head in the sand and self-righteously proclaim, "Not my kid!"

With this information, many parents may wonder if there is anything they can do (short of locking their kids in their room during their teen years) to influence their adolescents to make healthy choices regarding alcohol and drugs. We all know that, like the proverbial horse, you can lead a teen to water, and so on and so forth. However, if you provide your teen with knowledge and structure as opposed to dogmatically enforcing rules, you can help him/her make better choices. As Michael Riera (1995) writes, "Perhaps the most crucial factors are the conversations you have with your adolescent before usage ever becomes an issue and the example you set in your relationship to alcohol and drugs." Per Riera, parents should explicitly state their position on drugs and alcohol and discuss the possible consequences for violating these limits and agreements. Riera emphasizes that "the consequences should speak for themselves" so drug and alcohol use won't devolve into a power struggle between you and your teen. You also should acknowledge the reality regarding the difficulties of decision-making in the adolescent world. Be realistic. You shouldn't assume your teen will mess up, but don't be shocked if he/she does.

Education

Studies have shown that parental monitoring and involvement, as well as family cohesion, are important factors affecting adolescent academic success. Annunziata, et al. (2006) found that even moderate parental monitoring of adolescents from more cohesive families translates to more adolescent engagement in school. Parents should be involved in and aware of their adolescent's academic life, while still striving to maintain the level of autonomy their teen has already achieved. Involvement in your adolescent's education has been proven to be vital. In a 2014 study, Wang & Sheikh-Khalil found that "parent involvement in education predicted student academic success and mental health both directly and indirectly through behavioral and emotional engagement."

Riera (1995) stated that your goal as a parent should be to encourage learning as an enjoyable process throughout their lives. You can support this belief in your teens by asking open-ended, thoughtful questions concerning the process of your teens' learning. Involving yourself by asking these types of questions shows your teen the importance of learning and your interest in what he/she is learning. It also takes the focus away from being predominately about grades. As Riera cautions, "over the long run, parents pay dearly for driving their kids to study solely for the sake of grades." You should also discuss with your teen what your expectations are regarding how he/she manages the "job" of school, while helping him/her to develop personal goals and expectations.

Riera also suggests that parents set aside time each night for studying and reading. As he states, "the single most influential thing you can do to support learning is to practice what you preach." Having these types of established family routines have also been shown to support adolescent academic success. Roche & Ghazarian (2012) found that everyday family routines increased adolescent academic success.

It's ironic that many parents seem to remove themselves from active participation in their child's education as the child enters the middle and high school era. Research definitely indicates that parents' involvement unfortunately declines during this time frame. Nevertheless, it is prudent and critical that parents remain engaged. There are many areas in which parents should consider supporting their children while in secondary education or transitioning either to work or higher education. Teens may want their parents to "stay out of their business," but their education is our business. They may become so consumed with their social lives that education may not be a priority. Some teens may be in desperate need of help from others with their organization and priority setting–skills that reflect their difficulties with their executive functioning. It is our opinion that parents should provide support (some teens may need less guidance than others) in instituting a homework/study plan so that their teens stay on top of their responsibilities and work. This may mean that some parents need to help their teen focus on time management, organization, and perhaps adjust priorities. At times it may appear like a battlefront in the home, but in actuality we are helping our teens learn to develop a routine where they must balance both their social and academic lives. This may include limiting the teens' use of electronics so that they can stay focused on their schoolwork. Friends and associates who are classroom teachers have often commented that parental involvement is extremely important to a child's academic success. Awareness of a student's needs and problems may help not only the teacher but the student as well. Teachers are often overburdened with classroom loads and unaware of a student's need for understanding or acceptance. Parental contact with your teen's instructors can be crucial at this stage of his/her development. Sometimes the smallest bit of insight a teacher may have into a student's needs may yield great and unforeseen rewards.

It is imperative that we stay involved in talking with the school so that we know what is going on. Being involved at the school can be just as important for parents of a middle or high school student as a child in his/her primary years. Actually, middle school may be the most important time of your parenting since it is the time when most teens become sexually active. Teens may not understand what is happening to their bodies, but they may be more than willing to act upon these novel and unfamiliar feelings. Teens learn from the behavior and actions of their peers, but often the knowledge they pass along to one another has a tendency to be distorted. We can try and fly below the radar so as not to embarrass our teens, but we must let them know very clearly that we plan on being engaged. As parents, we need to set a standard of high expectations for our teens so that they don't disengage and take school too lightly. We need to be aware of what they're involved in and what they are doing so that we can help support them.

Sexuality

Sexuality is (and has probably always been) a rather uncomfortable topic between parents and teens. Some parents express concerns over social mores and health concerns (e.g., HIV/AIDS) that are different from parents' adolescent experience. Many are baffled and uncertain how to respond to those changes. In light of recent research about adolescent sexual activity, it is no wonder that parents are anxious about this aspect of raising an adolescent. A 2011 survey by the CDC revealed that over 47 percent of high school students had had sexual intercourse. That same year the report of another CDC survey determined that many adolescents are engaging in several more sexual behaviors other than just vaginal intercourse; almost half of the surveyed adolescents reported engaging in oral sex. One in ten of those surveyed had engaged in anal sex. Those are the facts, but before you begin your cry, "Get thee to a nunnery!" continue reading. As is the case in other aspects of their lives, parents can influence the choices adolescents make about sexual activity. Thus, no matter how awkward the conversation, you must talk to your kids about sex. Research has also shown that parents are constantly looking for ways to effectively discuss this topic with their teens. The concern over parental influence (especially in light of adolescent hormones) on teens' ideas regarding sexuality is evident. Parents are seeking ways not only to talk appropriately and pragmatically with their teens about sexuality, but also to impart parents' personal and/or religious views on the subject.

As Riera (1993) states, this is never a "value-free" topic—your personal and family values on this subject need to be communicated to your teen. In addition to this, teens must have "value-free" information: anatomy, development, birth control, and sexually transmitted infections. This should be delivered in tandem with discussions concerning relationships and emotions, as these are the elements that move teens towards deciding whether or not to be sexually active. You also have to realize that while you can earnestly impart these values and provide this information, in reality, you have little control over what happens. These are decisions your teens will be making on their own and at times when you are not present; hopefully they are guided by your conversations and the knowledge you impart to them. Finally, you must communicate to your teens that your love for them is more important than any uncomfortable feelings they are having. Even if this topic makes you squirm, your teen's health and well-being should supersede your lack of comfort.

Chores and teenagers

Although teenagers are at a stage where they're spreading their wings and stretching, they also need to be responsible for being participants and active contributors to the family household. Chores are just part of everyday living within a home and may range from basic housekeeping and laundry to taking care of the garden or helping prepare meals. Some parents view paying kids for chores as something that they shouldn't do because teens are members of the family and should contribute; others believe that children should be paid for contributing. This is a personal preference and no matter what your stance is regarding monetary compensation for chores, we believe that teenagers need to be held accountable and be involved in what goes on within a home.

What Teens Need to Successfully Adjust

If we could prepare a magic formula that morphed a child into a well-functioning adult, what ingredients would it include? In an article entitled "Counseling Parents of Adolescents," Leiman suggests four factors that seem to foster and help teenagers grow into effective young adults, rather than fostering rebellious youth. The four qualities that he highlighted that could be used in our formula are as follows:

(1) Providing quality family communication and attempting to understand what our teens are saying.
(2) Attempting to influence and enhance our teenager's self-image and self-worth.
(3) Promoting and teaching effective decision-making to our youth. Teaching our teens how to solve their own problems is truly a gift that they will need to survive. If we solve all of their problems they will not be able to do this on their own and will become too dependent on us. Finally, the last ingredient of the formula is the following:
(4) Effective discipline (p. 665), which in fact is one of the major tenets within this entire book. Dancing with our teens requires us to effectively lead; perhaps that in and of itself is a simple definition of effective discipline.

Each of these variables distinctly can make a strong contribution to enriching a teen's life. It seems only logical that good, effective communication (to be described in more detail later in this chapter) is a valuable technique to utilize with our teens. A summary of our simple formula is as follows: effective communication requires matching what we hear from our teens with appropriate verbal and non-verbal responses on our behalf. In addition, as parents, we must realize that we have the ability to enhance the self-image and resilience of our teen. In this way, we weatherproof our sons and daughters so that they will be capable of navigating through the storms in their lives.

Teaching decision-making skills is vital to function not only in the home but in life in general. As was highlighted just a moment ago, much of what is noted in the earlier chapters can be useful in directing our teens to make more appropriate life choices.

Building a More Resilient Teenager

Resiliency is our ability to keep on going in difficult periods. Teens that are resilient seem to bounce back from difficult outcomes and don't give up. Research on adolescent development seems to suggest that adolescents with high levels of parental support develop healthier levels of self-esteem and better social skills. Both of these variables promote resilience to the social pressures experienced by teens. Adolescents who experience more consistent regular forms of discipline are more resilient to peer influence. This resilience seems to make them less likely to subscribe to antisocial, less desirable choices.

In an executive summary of a recent Child Trends research brief relating to American teens, several points were noted about building a better teenager and what actually works. The paper highlighted four key elements that are crucial. We will briefly highlight each of them.

Relationships—specifically the relationships with their parents—seem to have a lot to do with successful adaptation in teens. It seems that the closer teens are with their parents, the more likely it is that they'll do better in school as well as in their social relations with friends. The second major ingredient pertains to our role as models. Parents who act as positive role models appear to have a healthy impact on detouring their teens' willingness to engage in risky behaviors.

Perhaps one of the most significant findings that was highlighted in this research brief related to our continued engagement with our teens. Contrary to the beliefs that teens distance themselves from their families, the research suggests that parents still need to remain active and positive in the lives of their teens, but, of course, in a different way. Parents who stay active also need to allow their adolescents to take on greater responsibility as they gain independence, and in doing so, begin to develop their own identity.

Parental perceptions of whether this is a great opportunity or a nightmare will also affect the way they interact with their adolescent. Adolescents need more space in which to grow than do younger children. It is perhaps not surprising that teens who are extended adult treatment (respect for mature decision-making, addressed as adults) are likely to respond in a mature fashion. We also need to give them the opportunity to make good choices. For example, some researchers (Templar 2013) assert that if you speak to your adolescent in a dignified and respectful manner, inquiring about his/her opinions (rather than speaking to them in a reactionary negative way) you will demonstrate to your adolescent that you have faith in the person he/she is becoming.

Finally, we must acknowledge that teenagers live in the moment and have a lot of trouble seeing past now (Wolfe 1991). Because they have only just started what they consider their adult life, they simply do not have the experience that comes with living. Thus, they lack one crucial piece of wisdom: experience. We must be patient with them and help them grow into their new lives and identities.

Suggested Tools to Parent Our Teenagers

A. Communication

The old saying that the pen is mightier than the sword is an appropriate metaphor as we introduce this next section of the chapter. We all have the capacity to listen to each other. Nevertheless, some of us seem to be better at connecting to others. Many intense conversations in families are stifled because various members may be lacking in effective communication. Parents who never truly listen during conversations and are very judgmental will have difficulty interacting productively with their teen. This causes barriers rather than paves pathways for change.

Many things seem to impact our ability to become effective listeners, ranging from not accurately hearing what's being said to misinterpreting a thought. Sometimes when we listen to people, they may not say what they are truly feeling, and we need to probe more deeply to find out what they are really trying to say. The unfortunate part is that our inadequacy or discomfort in communication can derail effective connections.

Perhaps one of the greatest steps to dancing effectively with teens is the importance of being a good listener. We need to let our teens know that we will listen to them. Wolf (1991), in his book *Get Out of My Life,* stresses, "…Listening means listening, not giving advice. But if parents say this, they must mean it." Wolf also stresses the importance of communicating important values and traits to your teen through your actions, not just words. Listening may sound easy enough to do, but you'd be surprised at how often people really don't pay any attention to what the other person is trying to say. Being a good listener is more than simply not interrupting the speaker. It's also more than just hearing the words of the speaker. It's hearing *and* trying to understand what is being said.

As Stephenson, et al. (2005) found, parents who valued communication with their children were also more likely to balance limit setting, warmth and expression, and autonomy granting in the parent–child relationship. All of these are vital aspects of the aforementioned authoritative parenting style that has proven effective time and again. This open approach to communication can support a stronger family bond, and many researchers found that adolescents are less likely to use alcohol or drugs when they felt a strong family bond (McGee, 1992; Lattimore, Vischer, & Linster, 1995; Duncan, Tildesley, Duncan, & Hopps, 1995; Segal & Fairchild, 1996; Sokol-Katz, Dunham, & Zimmerman, 1997).

Congruent Communication

Haim Ginott, a child psychologist, is perhaps the most prolific advocate espousing the value of listening and talking to our teens. His greatest contribution to child/parent relationships was something he classified as congruent communication. The emphasis of this form of communication was that it is "harmonious, authentic and where words fit feelings" (79). Congruent communication addresses the behavioral situation on hand by clarifying the feelings addressed. This could prove particularly effective with a difficult teen with whom we're dealing. Congruent communication does not put the teen on the defense because we are not promoting an argument. In essence, congruent communication focuses on situations, not a teen's character or personality. It focuses on the behavior of today and not of yesterday. Focusing on the past often becomes a source of many arguments. Of course, for this strategy to work, the parent must be able to exercise emotional control. This can be difficult especially in extreme situations and can possibly push the limits of a parent's ability to remain calm.

Utilizing congruent communication teaches parents not to preach or impose guilt on their child. Rather, parents should attempt to confer a sense of dignity and help their child make good decisions. Sane messages are when parents address a teen's behavior rather than his/her character. In this way, the problem is dealt with rather than parenting a subjective view of the child. "Empathy not only matters; it is the foundation of effective parenting" (Gottman, 1996, p. 35). Communication and the empathy incorporated in our interactions are perhaps among the greatest strengths that parents bring to their interactions with their teens. As Gottman notes, we need to become "emotion coaches" and listen to what our children are trying to tell us.

Congruent communication allows parents to convey a sense of mutual respect and dignity in their interactions. Typically, utilizing communication in this manner will engage teens and encourage involvement, focusing our strong attention on the present rather than on the past.

Reflective Listening

In a book on attention and learning disorders that we wrote several years ago, we had a section where we described reflective listening. The approach is defined as attending and responding with sensitivity to both verbal and non-verbal messages coming from the child. In order to more effectively communicate as parents, we need to learn to accurately respond not only to the content of what a child is saying, but also to the message. With a growing acceptance of reflective listening, parents are beginning to realize that when responding to a child's feelings they need not only to be aware of what the child is saying verbally, but also to pay attention to what the child is expressing non-verbally. One can learn a great deal about the intentions of another by looking at facial expressions or posture. Sometimes, the words our teens are saying may not match their non-verbal actions, which could present a challenge for parents.

In order to develop responsive statements, as parents, we will have to integrate two components. In the first part of the response, we need to formulate a statement that integrates what we believe the child feels. We must do this by using a simple, "you feel ______" formula. To develop a more comprehensive vocabulary, parents may want to practice developing five or ten feeling words to enhance their ability to express what a child may be feeling. Table 1 provides a more extensive list of feeling words. You are encouraged to review the list and begin practicing using some of the terms.

Following identifying how the child is feeling, parents can integrate the second component in this communication, which is to connect with what the child is saying. The content explains the teen's reasons for the feelings and behavior. Reflective listening is at its best when you respond accurately, thus encouraging teens to talk in more detail as they now feel understood. When you're incorrect, teens will often correct you because they appreciate the genuineness within the conversation. Another skill that should be applied to reflective listening is paraphrasing. Paraphrasing what someone says helps put into our own words what you've heard from his/her statement. This restating of what your child says can prove incredibly useful in communicating well with your teen. Paraphrasing may begin with a phrase as simple as, "Let me see if I understood you correctly."

It is evident that one thing that blocks teens from communicating is our apparent deafness to what they are trying to say. It is often challenging to discern exactly what is troubling the teen, since many teens are not fully able to reflect upon (or understand) the deeper issues facing them. They also have difficulty clearly articulating their feelings about these issues to their parents. We must mean what we say and follow through with what we are going to do. Your teen needs to realize that you're going to be consistent and you're going to resolve issues in a fair and thoughtful manner.

Many people often find it difficult to put into words *exactly* what they're trying to say. No two people think and speak in *exactly* the same terms or phrases. Because of this, we may intend to convey one message but the listener may hear an altogether different message. This occurs frequently when parents and adolescents get together. They simply don't speak the same language. The best way to overcome this obstacle, however, is a procedure called "checking out." When your teenager says something to you, you may want to repeat his message back to him *in your own words* and ask him if that's what he meant. In short, "check out" with him whether or not you fully understood what he's just said. This procedure takes very little time and effort, but it prevents a lot of misunderstanding and hard feelings. Of course, being a good listener in no way guarantees that you're going to like what you hear, but at least you'll know for sure what the speaker intends. Phrases like, "If I understand you correctly, you mean ________," and, "Is this what you are trying to say?" are valuable skills in a parent's repertoire.

Table 1 provides some useful guidelines on how you can learn to apply reflective listening at home. To become more effective with these skills, we encourage you to practice your moves so you can more gracefully communicate with your youngster.

Table 1
The Delicate Dance of Conversation:
How to Become a Better Communicator with Your Teen
Utilizing Reflective Listening

Introduction: The importance of Parent-Teen communication with reflective listening

What is reflective listening?

Reflective listening is:

- **a)** Hearing *and* understanding what the speaker is communicating (both verbally and non-verbally)
- **b)** Responding to the speaker by reflecting his/her thoughts and feelings with things such as tone of voice, body posture, and gestures

Why should parents use reflective listening with their teens?

One reason is to help understand what their child is trying to convey. Other benefits of reflective listening are the following:

- **a)** To allow your teen to feel heard and understood/listened to
- **b)** To provide feedback to your teen on how what he/she said was interpreted/came across
- **c)** To help the parent stay focused during the conversation

When should parents apply reflective listening?

- **a)** When a parent is experiencing a problem or difficult situation
- **b)** When there is a need for conflict management, problem-solving, etc.
- **c)** When leading family or group discussions

Ways to Communicate Effectively

How to conduct a reflective conversation with your teen: steps to follow

a) What do parents need to know about reflecting skills?
   Reflecting skills are the "checking out" process. You should respond to the content and feelings of what the other has expressed.
   a. Reflect or express to the other person the essence of what he/she has expressed (verbally and non-verbally)
   b. Summarize larger segments of what has been said/interpreted
   c. Use when a significant segment of communication is heard

b) Reflective listening: steps to implement
   Acknowledgment response: Simple, brief (verbal or non-verbal) responses to show that listener is following conversation, such as uh-huh, yeah, I see, right, sounds good, etc.

   Repeating/rephrasing: Listener repeats, with similar terminology, what speaker stated. This is a simple formula to follow—"You feel ____________(feeling word) because ____________________(behavior, what actually occurred)." You could end the sentence with an additional insight, which would strengthen your response. Often, after hearing a reflective comment, a teen may be more apt to continue the conversation.

   Reflecting content/paraphrasing: Listener makes complete restatement in which speaker's meaning is inferred.

   Reflection of feeling: Listener emphasizes emotional aspects of communication through feeling statements—deepest form of listening. This is very critical. We, as parents, may benefit from learning more appropriate feeling words (a list is provided at the end of this table).

   Reflecting meanings: Reflecting feelings and content that the teen has expressed. This is crucial and is probably one of the greatest benefits of reflective listening.

Summarizing: Condensing and summarizing what the speaker has said. Asking open-ended questions rather than closed-ended questions.

"I" messages vs. "You" Messages

a) Parents should use **"I" messages** rather than **"you" messages**.
b) "I" message example: "I am very upset."
"I" messages point out what you're feeling as opposed to pointing blame.
c) "You" message example: "You are being very unfair."
d) Use laconic language. "Laconic" means short and to the point.

Practice example: Below are examples for you to observe "I" vs. "you" communication and reflective listening.

Teen comes home late after curfew.

Parent "I" message: I feel ____________(feeling word) when you___________(behavior) because___________________

Teen is failing all his classes because he is playing with his electronics.

Parent "I" message: I feel ____________(feeling word) when you___________(behavior) because___________________

Teen fails to complete any of her chores while the parent went out.

Parent "I" message: I feel ____________(feeling word) when you___________(behavior) because___________________

What are attending skills?

Attending is giving your physical and psychological attention to another person in communication.

What are some typical attending skills?

e) Non-verbal skills

a. These are used to communicate without words that there is rapport between you and the other

b. Eye contact

c. Gestures

d. Environment

e. Interested silence

Feeling Words

Example for parents to use great feeling words

http://www.psychpage.com/learning/library/assess/feelings.html

Pleasant Feelings			
OPEN	HAPPY	ALIVE	GOOD
UNDERSTANDING	GREAT	PLAYFUL	CALM
CONFIDENT	GAY	COURAGEOUS	PEACEFUL
RELIABLE	JOYOUS	ENERGETIC	AT EASE
EASY	LUCKY	LIBERATED	COMFORTABLE
LOVE	INTERESTED	POSITIVE	STRONG
LOVING	CONCERNED	EAGER	IMPULSIVE
CONSIDERATE	AFFECTED	KEEN	FREE
AFFECTIONATE	FASCINATED	EARNEST	SURE
SENSITIVE	INTRIGUED	INTENT	CERTAIN

Difficult/Unpleasant Feelings			
ANGRY	DEPRESSED	CONFUSED	HELPLESS
IRRITATED	LOUSY	UPSET	INCAPABLE
ENRAGED	DISAPPOINTED	DOUBTFUL	ALONE
HOSTILE	DISCOURAGED	UNCERTAIN	PARALYZED
INSULTING	ASHAMED	INDECISIVE	FATIGUED
INDIFFERENT	AFRAID	HURT	SAD
INSENSITIVE	FEARFUL	CRUSHED	TEARFUL
DULL	TERRIFIED	TORMENTED	SORROWFUL
NONCHALANT	SUSPICIOUS	DEPRIVED	PAINED
NEUTRAL	ANXIOUS	PAINED	GRIEF

"I" Messages

"I" messages were coined by Thomas Gordon as a method of assertively communicating your intentions without putting people on the defensive. They are messages that describe the behavior that we're concerned with, and the feelings that we have, but don't threaten a teenager. "You" messages, on the other hand, focus more directly on the person and often get poorer responses. For example, listen to how the following sentences sound and how they could be interpreted.

"You're always late."

"You do this wrong."

"You make me angry."

Traditionally, when teenagers hear these statements, the effect is often negative and may cause them to turn off. An "I" message softens the blow of a difficult conversation, but gets the point across. For example, the following demonstrates how to put together an "I" message for a teen that comes in late. "I worry when you don't come in on time because I'm not sure where you are. Please follow the directions." The formula for an "I" message is the following:

I feel (put in the feeling word)

when (the behavior that causes the feeling).

What you would like the teen to do in the future.

Arguing

The simplest suggestion that can be given is avoid the small battles; prioritizing issues in order of importance and relevance is important.

We suggest that a parent should avoid punishing when he/she is angry with his/her child. Reactive responses are often not the most viable options. It's best to avoid arguments when a calm mind isn't present. A second suggestion is to avoid time lapses in administering punishments and also be consistent. The longer you wait to respond, the more insignificant the punishment. You also need to try to deliver similar consequences for similar challenges. If a parent threatens punishment, he/she needs to carry it out if the child continues to express undesired behavior. Often, when sucked into an argument, some parents select the most unreasonable punishments. For example, how many parents have said, "You are grounded for life"? We believe that the punishment should never exceed the undesired behavior and should be only as long as really necessary. Effective and positive parenting is about teaching, supporting, and guiding our teen, not just demanding his/her obedience. Teens must see that we are invested in them and deeply care.

The greatest challenge when arguments occur is that they often change the climate within the home. Arguments make people feel edgy and consequently, at times, it isn't only the teen that gets into difficulty in terms of punishment. We need to make our best efforts not to take out our frustrations on other family members. Finally, as discussed earlier, when trying to solve conflict, focus on the problem. "Ginott emphasizes that criticizing the action rather than the child will preserve the child's self-esteem and lessen the chances that the undesired behavior will occur." (Leiman, p. 667).

Problem ownership—problem-solving

"It is best not to volunteer verbal remedies. Fix that. Instead, we let our teenager use his own initiative to deal with life situations. Acknowledging the difficulty and waiting for his suggestions allows him to assert his will and exercise his autonomy."–54

From Ginott, Teacher and Child

Often, parents find themselves in situations where they dictate to their teen what needs to occur, rather than collaborating so that the teen is invested in the solution. Now that we've talked about communication somewhat, we thought it would be really helpful to discuss ways that one could help a child/teenager solve a problem and reach a viable solution. It's interesting that when a person owns a solution, that individual is more willing to put it into action. The following section briefly identifies some simple steps that you can take as a model to teach your teen problem-solving. However, before we discuss problem clarification let's talk a little bit about who owns the problem first.

Problem ownership is especially crucial because sometimes we may try to institute a solution to a problem that will have little meaning to the youngster because the problem isn't his/hers to begin with. If a teen owns the issue, we can be supportive, but shouldn't take on the problem as our own. For example, let's say the teen is having an argument with a friend and the teen is feeling bad. We should leave the problem in the teen's hands to solve, but be there to help support him/her rather than just giving our opinions on how to solve it. The problem then becomes his/hers and we act only to support the teen.

Dealing with a teen is quite simply like peeling an onion. We need to look more deeply to understand what that problem is and how it needs to be solved. Typically, the four stages of problem-solving include identifying and clarifying what the problem is, followed by the possible solutions. Once a solution is selected, we could help our teen monitor the plan that was selected. Once completed, the teen can begin to evaluate whether the option selected worked or not and how it could be improved.

As parents, it is important to establish clear guidelines with your teen. I always look at rules and structure as almost like putting bumpers on a bowling alley. The metaphor of bumpers seems to work very appropriately with this example; using the bumper metaphor allows a teen to be successful with minimal accommodations. Raising teens requires parents to recognize that rules are the basic element in any given day. The rules and guidelines provide reasonable accommodations (bumpers for teens to use), so they will not get into trouble (or in a bowling metaphor, will not throw gutter balls). Having vague expectations can cause friction between you and your teen, and you may respond in an over-reactive manner. Rules need to be based on what you expect a person to do. As a parent, you need to be not only consistent and clear, but also focused on the expected behavior and what you mean exactly. For example, if you tell your teen to come home at 10:00 p.m., does that mean no later than 10:00 p.m.? Could it mean if the child comes in at 10:15 p.m. that will be acceptable? Is it acceptable to be late some of the time or never acceptable at all? We need to be very clear as to what the rules are and how they will be enforced. By making sure that the rule is related to rewards and consequences, parents identify to the teen what is expected. So many of the things that we've talked about earlier about consistency, making the behavior relate to the reinforcer, or the punishment methods are still in place.

Rules for teens

We believe that meaningful rules for teens require teen involvement in drafting and implementation of said rules. Receiving their input and helping them problem-solve increases the likelihood that rules will be followed. Nevertheless, at times, it is totally appropriate for parents to let their teens know that certain issues aren't negotiable. On the other hand, getting the teen's commitment may result in stronger compliance. We need to realize that it is one thing to get compliance but another thing to get their commitment to follow through. As parents, we should strive for more than mere compliance. Obedience in the absence of deep commitment is transitory and rarely results in transformative behavior.

It's equally important for us to recognize that rules commonly need to be adapted. And that means over time, when a rule is not necessary any more, we either modify or delete it. Scaffolding what our expectations are allows us to move back and forth so we again provide the most accurate supports that are needed. Teenagers need to be able to fly freely, but we want to make sure that when they're flying, they're flying safely and with guidance that will get them to the place that they need to be.

Rules have to be fair. When we talk about fair rules, the discussion allows a teenager to give input. When you're making the rules, some professionals recommend that you write down the rule, and that you write down the consequences so that there's no gray in what the expectations are.

Let's summarize the guidelines for rules.
They need to be clear,
They need to be concise,
And they need to be non-confrontational.

When a rule is implemented, all need to recognize that we're not going to fight over this; we're going to just follow this through. Perhaps one of the greatest challenges in parenting teenagers is that we tend often to get ourselves into arguments with our teens, and that's something that we need to avoid. We need to stick with what the guideline is, and in fairness, work through the entire outcome. In essence, as parents of teenagers, we need to learn to control only what we *can* control. We need to realize that certain things may not be worth the battle that will be set up for us, if we try to fight it.

Suggestions for Avoiding Conflict

When interacting with teens, parents should keep in mind the many useful ideas and insights that can be put in place. Now that we have discussed communication and problem-solving, let's synthesize some points that seem to be easy to put into place. Although these are our own thoughts, many mental health leaders who have contributed to parenting, such as William Glasser, Haim Ginott, Rudolf Dreikurs, and Thomas Gordon, have influenced our beliefs. It's important for us to focus on the present issues and avoid focusing on the past. Many arguments usually begin and are accelerated when the past is brought up, especially when it is used as evidence for disappointment. We believe that it makes much more sense to focus on the here and now. As much as possible, try to stay away from criticizing and blaming our teens when trying to solve a present challenge.

As we discussed earlier, we all could use an internal gauge to help control our reactive behavior. All of us have had occasions where we regret the way we responded to our children. We recommend that whenever you feel frustrated, simply walk away; it may be more useful to walk away and restrain your emotions rather than saying or doing something that you will regret later.

As a rule of thumb, do not impose your own will and thoughts on your teen. You need to recognize that it may not be worth all of the battles that you may put into this to get your point across. It's really important that we treat our teens with the sense of respect that we, in turn, would like to receive from them. Although we see our teens as our children, and although they may act like they are immature, they're no longer children. We need to give them the opportunity to earn that level of respect.

Parenting a teen can be stressful at times, but try to keep everything in perspective. Trying to stay positive whenever possible is a valuable asset. A golden rule to follow is to be non-judgmental in your actions and avoid put-downs and negativity.

Staying collected and positive helps reduce stress and improves relationships within the home. A simple smile or a gentle pat on the back can really help relieve a situation. Giving your teen a choice and avoiding being an authoritarian are also crucial because allowing a teen to be an engaged partner in decision-making will get him/her more committed.

The last suggestion we would like to give is not getting bogged down with accepting excuses. We need to get children to learn to be accountable for what they're doing, and we should be patient and supportive of their actions.

Behavioral contracts

Many of the techniques that were discussed in the earlier chapters could be applied with teens, but behavioral contracts seem to be more easily integrated with teens and parents. A behavioral contract is a written agreement that could be formulated and developed between a parent and his/her teen. The document, in essence, specifies both the behavior, which is required by the teen in addition to the consequences, and the rewards that will be implemented contingent on following the guidelines of the contract.

Contracting is based on good practices of behaviorism, but it can be a very humanistic approach. As a procedure, as I mentioned, it works really well with older children, because it gives them a chance to negotiate what the consequences and rewards could be. Furthermore, this procedure is quite effective with those who are capable and want to take an active role in collaborating, which we believe is an important set of standards for teens. Simply, a contract is a clear articulation of what is expected of the teen and how he/she will be reinforced. Again, it is important to encourage a commitment for change from the teen so that he/she will be more motivated.

Contracts should encourage and recognize successive approximations of the goal that we want to establish. In this way the teen will experience success and be motivated to work towards the final outcome of the expected behavior. It has always been understood that the more involved teens are in solving their problems, the more involved they are in generating the solutions.

The following are the basic guidelines of how parents should develop a contract with their teens:

1. The contract that's being developed should be reward/performance-based and the rewards should be given immediately when the contract is met.
2. Contracts should be organized to gradually develop the desired behavior that is expected. It seems ridiculous to quickly expect dramatic changes in a teen, and a contract should recognize this. For example, a contract to modify a notoriously late teen's behavior would specify that if the teen comes in four out of five days on time or within a certain time limit, he/she will earn a reward. Consequently, we and our teen become more focused on the goal at hand.
3. Contracts should provide frequent rewards in small increments. This helps the teen eventually incorporate the behavior into his/her daily life, as well as enhance how it will be maintained after the contract is removed. If we can help our teen recognize that he/she is changing for his/her own good, he/she is more likely to comply.
4. Rewards should only be presented contingent upon the behavior actually occurring.
5. The contract should always be written in the positive and clearly understood by all parties involved. We suggest a written and dated contract before implementation so that all are aware of the guidelines.

6. The contract should be developed fairly for both the child and the parent. (It would be unfortunate if those responsible for developing the contract were not being honest with the other party.) Furthermore, although it's expected that the contract's major purpose is to motivate the teen externally, we want to genuinely respect the integrity of that teenager.
7. Contracts should be negotiated as well as agreed upon by all parties.
8. The final element that we believe a contract should have is clarity of purpose: clearly defined rewards, openly agreed-upon times for evaluation and re-negotiation.

In most cases, contracts are usually not effective on their own in controlling dangerous and destructive behaviors but really work well in helping youngsters agree to an act that they're working towards.

Sample Contract

Child's name.

Parent's name.

Date of Agreement. (Contract Begins on ___________(Date) and ends on ___________(Date). The contract will be reviewed on ___________(Date).

If ____
_______________________________________ (clearly identify the expected behavior, as well as where and when that behavior is to occur) is to be accomplished by _________________(Date), then you will earn the following _______________________________
____________(the agreed-upon reward).
Child's signature ______________________

Parent's signature______________________

Date__________________________

Final Thoughts

The dance during the roller coaster years can be challenging to learn but easily mastered if you are open to change. A sailor once told us a metaphor about sailing that seems apropos as we conclude this chapter. He noted that when he used to sail there were times that the wind wasn't cooperating and the sailing that day wasn't as enjoyable. That used to upset him until he realized that "you cannot always change the wind, but you can adjust your sails." When adjusting your sails, you still get to where you need to go. Parenting tweens/teens may require adjustments to our previous strategies and our acceptance that our children are growing up. Sure, there are differences, but that is what makes parenting so interesting. As Hodding Carter Jr. once elegantly pointed out, "There are two lasting bequests we can give our children. One is roots. The other is wings." During the teen years, our teens are beginning to try to fly on their own. Patience, guidance, and support are what they need from us as they transition to more independence through this challenging era.

References

Aitchison, R., & Eimers, R. (1977). *Effective parents/responsible children.* New York: McGraw-Hill.

American Psychiatric Association. (2002). *Developing adolescents: A reference for professionals.* Washington, DC: Author.

American Psychological Association. *Communication tips for parents.* Retrieved from https://www.apa.org/helpcenter/communication-parents.aspx

Annunziata D., Hogue A., Faw, L. & Liddle, H. (2006). Family functioning and school success in at-risk, inner-city adolescents. *Journal of Youth and Adolescence,* 35(1), 105–113.

Attaway, N., & Bry, B. (2004). Parenting style and black adolescents' academic achievement. *Journal of Black Psychology,* 30, 229–247.

Brooks, R., & Goldstein, S. (2001). *Raising Resilient Children: Fostering strength, hope and optimism in your children.* Chicago: Contemporary Books.

Center for Disease Control and Prevention. (2011). *Sexual behavior, sexual attraction, and sexual identity in the united states: Data from the 2006–2008 national survey of family growth* (DHHS Publication No. PHS 2011–1250). Washington, DC: U.S. Government Printing Office.

Commendador, K. (2011). The relationship between maternal parenting style, female adolescent decision making, and contraceptive use. *Journal of the American Academy of Nurse Practitioners, 23, 561–572.*

Dweck, C. (2007). The perils and promise of praise. *Educational Leadership*, 34–39.

Elliott, S. & Aseltine, E. (2013). Raising teenagers in hostile environments: How race, class, and gender matter for mothers' protective carework. *Journal of Family Issues*, 34:719.

Feiler, B. (2013). *The secrets of happy families: Improve your mornings, rethink family dinner, fight smarter, go out and play, and much more.* New York: HarperCollins.

Ginott H. (1972) *Between parent and teenagers. New York: Macmillan.*

Gottman, J. M. (1996). *Raising an emotionally intelligent child.* New York: Simon & Schuster.

Hale, W., et al. (2013). Is adolescent generalized anxiety disorder a magnet for negative parental interpersonal behaviors? *Depression and Anxiety, 41, 849–856.*

Howard, B. J. (2010). Ask Dr. Howard. *Working Mother*, 33(5), 92.

Hurt, T., Brody, G., Murry, V., Berkel, C. & Chen, Y. (2013). Elucidating parenting processes that influence adolescent alcohol use: A qualitative inquiry. *Journal of Adolescent Research*, 28:3.

Jenkins, J., Meunier, J., & Wade, M. (2012). Mothers' differential parenting and children's behavioural outcomes: Exploring the moderating role of family and social context. *Infant and Child Development, 21, 107–133.*

Kastner, L. & Wyatt, J. (2009). *Getting to calm: Cool-headed strategies for parenting teens and tweens.* Seattle: Parent Map.

Krysan, M., Moore, K. A., & Zill, N. (1990). *Research on successful families.* U.S. Department of Health and Human Services.

Kurz, D. (2002). Caring for teenage children. *Journal of Family Issues*, 23:748.

Leiman, A. H., & Strasburger, V. C. (1985). Counseling parents of adolescents. *Pediatrics,* 76(4), 664.

Londergan, B. (2008) *The agony and the agony: Raising your teenager without losing your mind.* New York: Da Capo Press.

McKinney, C. & Milone, M. (2012). Parental and late adolescent psychopathology: Mothers may provide support when needed most. *Child Psychiatry & Human Development, 43, 747–760.*

McNeely, C. A., & Barber, B. K. (2010). How do parents make adolescents feel loved? Perspectives on supportive parenting from adolescents in 12 cultures. *Journal of Adolescent Research*, 25(4), 601–631.

Moore, K. & Zaff, J. (2002). Building a better teenager: A summary of "what works" in adolescent development. *Child Trends*, 57, 1–5.

Nowinski, J. (2007). *The identity trap: Saving our teens from themselves.* New York, NY: AMACOM.

Riera, M. (1995). *Uncommon sense for parents with teenagers.* Berkeley: Celestial Arts.

Roche, K. & Ghazarian, S. (2012). The value of family: Routines for the academic success of vulnerable adolescents. *Journal of Family Issues*, 33(7), 874–897.

Sachs, Brad E. (2001). *The good enough child.* New York, NY: Harper Collins.

Sorkhabi, N. (2013). Conflict emergence and adaptiveness of normative parent-adolescent conflicts: Baumrind's socialization theory and cognitive social domain theory. In Larzelere, R., Morris, A. S., Harrist, A. W. (Eds.), Authoritative parenting: Synthesizing nurturance and discipline for optimal child development (pp. 137–161). Washington, D.C.: American Psychological Association.

Templar, R. (2013). *The rules of parenting* (2nd. Ed.). Edinburgh: Pearson.

Tewari, N. (1998). Parachute kids in southern California: The educational experience of Chinese children in transnational families. *Educational Policy, 12(6), 682–704.*

Warr, M. (2006). The tangled web: Delinquency, deception, and parental attachment. *Youth Adolescence, 36, 607–622.*

Wang, M. & Sheikh-Khalil, S. (2014). Does parental involvement matter for student achievement and mental health in high school? *Child Development*, 85(2), 610–625.

Wolf, A. E. (1991). *Get out of my life, but first could you drive me and Cheryl to the mall? A parent's guide to the new teenager.* New York, NY: The Noonday Press.

CHAPTER 8

Enhancing Life within the Family: Recipes to Make Home Life More Meaningful and Enjoyable

The boys have moved from California, and are now living on the east coast and Colorado. Whenever the family comes together, it's always time for reminiscing and reconnecting. We just had one of those occasions last weekend. We all sat around and talked about the days gone by. We laughed a lot, especially at stories where Mom and Dad were the butt of the joke. A favorite related to "Mom's rules." Basically, in our home no one (even a dignitary) was able to eat in the family room. It was like committing a cardinal sin, especially if you got caught. The boys laughed about the times when one of them got caught and how it was dealt with. Well, one of the evenings over that weekend, we lived "Mom's rules" once again. After eating dessert, we left the table to sit in the family room. I didn't join them when they were walking off because I wasn't done. The boys turned around and looked at me and said, "Dad, aren't you coming?" I replied, "In a few minutes when I finish what I am eating." They both looked at me, smiled and at the same moment in unison, said, "Mom's rules still live, huh?"

Family rituals and family activities have been celebrated for thousands of years. "Mom's rules" is a perfect example of a family ritual that is still remembered and joyfully celebrated.

Although there is a great deal of joy that can be gained in family interactions, life within a family can be quite complicated. We wouldn't lie and say that life is a bed of roses. There are times we can all feel supreme happiness while on other occasions we may ponder ultimate dejection. We wish there were a formula or recipe for perfect family living, but we must realize what is perfect for one family may not feel natural for another. Family dynamics are unique to each family, and it is not possible to delineate a standard template for all humanity, independent of cultural mores. There are, however, many ways that one can make life more meaningful for everyone involved. Building a stronger family takes a commitment to making family life a priority. Strong families just don't appear or materialize out of some insubstantial fabric, they occur because we make family time important. We give it substance, and what we put into it is what we can get out of it.

If a family elixir really could be made, we are certain that it would be patented and sold universally. The simple answer to our quandary is that having meaningful opportunities within our homes means that we have to have a strong commitment to employ ideas that can work. Most of these ideas don't require wealth but rather a commitment to be closer to one's children. We need to get our hands dirty and prioritize our efforts. Our thoughts have already been amplified in our writings throughout the earlier chapters. Happier families learn to co-exist because there is not only a commitment but also a built-in system of consistent discipline that is dispensed with fairness. On the other hand, there are so many other ingredients that can enhance family life, including daily family rituals, having fun with one's children (including having pets in the home), family meetings, and strategies to diffuse conflict. We will discuss several of these issues in this chapter. Chapter 9 will continue this discussion but focus on promoting unity within our homes with sections on family companion animals, family leisure, and our children's extracurricular activities.

Family Routines and Rituals

Rituals can range from unique family interactions that enhance familial connectedness to the very mundane encounters which solidify family ties.

Viere (2001) once stated that rituals are powerful organizers and in many ways help families socialize their children in a cultural manner. When most people think of rituals, the first things that pops into their heads are Sunday dinners, family movie or game night, or even reading bedtime stories. Others may consider routines at dinner, like having a moment to share an important part of everyone's day, or taking yearly trips to the same destination. Our family routines and rituals help us impart our family values and traditions. They put our mark on the family and help us become a unit.

In the Fine household, we had many of these traditions that I think helped us feel more connected. We had game nights and a special evening designated for everyone to have a turn at preparing and a cooking a meal. Some were yummy and scrumptious, while others didn't work quite as well. Nevertheless, they always proved to be great fun. I always think back to days when the clean-up took longer than the preparation and eating of the dinners. I didn't even realize that we had so many utensils in the kitchen.

Perhaps a ritual that portrayed our family well (especially when the boys were young) was when the boys had friends sleep over. Only in the "Fine household" would a sleep over turn into a major extravaganza. It began just before everybody settled in to go to bed and a story would be introduced about a mystical animal that would visit you in your dreams and wreak havoc while you were sleeping. The ritual typically got everyone to sleep quickly. Let's reminisce for a moment:

Weekends in the Fine home were always busy times. Hockey had always been played and most often teammates were invited over for an evening of games, eating and hanging out, followed by sleeping over. Every evening ended somewhat the same. The Tadger story would be told. The Tadger is a mystical animal that is a combination of a tiger and a badger. Both my wife and I learned the story when we worked at camps, but we adapted it a little bit for our own children. The story was simple. It was about this animal named Tadger that was just a very fun-loving, mischief-making creature. While people would be sleeping, Tadger would sneak into your home and perform lighthearted pranks that would bring smiles to your faces. Our job wasn't to catch Tadger in the act, but to allow him to do his thing and to awaken the next morning to witness the pranks. Sometimes we would find remnants of things that would be out of place to realize that he had come. However, you always knew he graced your home, if he left a print mark on your face (typically a little lipstick).

The original Tadger story typically was shared to young campers at a campsite. A lot more natural havoc could occur in the great outdoors, especially to the food that was designated for morning breakfast. It was breakfast items like small cereal boxes, bananas, doughnuts, and little trinkets of food that could be really toyed with. Typically, when the children would awaken, they would find their breakfast hanging from the tress, some of the clothing scattered over the campsite, and they would all find a small Tadger marking on their face. In our home, we had to modify some of the Tadger pranks, but the mark on the face was always a highlight! As the boys grew older, I knew they realized that the Tadger wasn't real but that it was an extravaganza, a ritual that was part of our family which they loved to celebrate. As they aged, I think it was just more for fun; could they catch us in the middle of the night setting up the fantasy, or would we get away with it and watch their faces as they would awaken to witness all the havoc?

Families that learn to play with each other and enjoy themselves are families that may function better. It takes hard work, but we believe it is worth the effort. Over fifty years ago, a seminal paper by Bossard and Boyle (1950) was written focusing on family rituals. Although the paper is very much dated by our standards, their insights about the importance of these rituals are very consistent to our lifestyles of today. Through detailed analyses of diaries, interviews, and family memorabilia, they concluded that rituals (such as family chores, eating dinner together, bedtimes, etc.) are powerful organizers of family life. These rituals help support the stability of any family and particularly seem to support them during times of stress and transition.

Many would agree that family routines seem to help stabilize families. Even requiring our children to complete chores offers us an opportunity to teach our children responsibility and new skills. We need to look beyond the requested act and realize that completing chores helps build our children's sense of responsibility, commitment, and character. Children also learn by actions, so make sure that what you say to them is what you mean and do. You help them realize that a given expectation is that they follow through. Often, routines help create a sense of togetherness. We should not focus on perfectionism, especially when first introducing chores to young children, but rather the completion of the task and maintaining a positive attitude in finishing the task. We need to show our children that every person within a family has a job and that the children, too, are fulfilling their roles. As parents, we also need to fairly disperse assignments so that children aren't unfairly given excessive chores. They need to be given reasonable options that are developmentally commensurate for their age. Research conducted on families seems to agree that children who have responsibilities in their homes seem to be more adjusted later in life. In a study at the University of Minnesota, researchers found that the best predictor of young adult success was whether the subjects participated in household chores by the age of four.

Interestingly, if a young adult did not start doing chores until later in his/her life, the same positive effects weren't visible.

Family Dinners

Dinnertime is a fantastic opportunity for teaching and learning. So much can be learned at a dinner, especially if you listen and reduce distractions. One thing that has been waning over the years has been eating as a family or eating without disruptions. When our children were younger we had a rule that the TV was off during the meals. We all have enough distractions in our lives throughout the day that having a meal together could be just that: food in the company of one's family. It is a routine that seems to be losing its popularity because of the busy schedules we lead today, but it is one that we should be reluctant to lose. Research over the years has found mealtime to be especially helpful on promoting family well-being (Fulkerson et al. 2006). It is our opinion that the rituals established at family meals can enhance family connectedness and unity.

It isn't actually the meal that is the important part; it is coming together and being a family. Mealtime discussions can be integrated into the lifestyles of even busy families who have hectic work schedules and tremendous extracurricular commitments that conflict with typical dinnertimes. Families can make other options work in other ways, like having early morning breakfasts or incorporating evening snacks or desserts. The most important aspect must be to make the time to talk and to be together. To do otherwise fragments the family unit.

At these meals if we take the time to listen to each other, we can learn if our child is having a great day or is experiencing some challenges. It can also be an opportunity for family members to learn more about each other. With proper questions, we can discover a great deal about each other. Finally, Farris (2013) points out that having family meals allows for the children to develop an "intergenerational self" where "they know they belong to something bigger than themselves" (p. 42). We agree with this point of view and believe that during family meals, it is important that children and adults have the opportunity to hear stories of the past and learn about their family's history.

Is there a formula to encourage more dynamic family conversation? We believe that the most critical part is to try to have the child engaged and become an active participant. If the child has difficulty generating conversation, perhaps periodically have themes for conversations at the table or an idea jar from which topics could be pulled. There are many ideas that could be generated and one's personal preference should lead the way. There are even games that can be purchased which contain lists of great questions that could help orchestrate a fun and revealing conversation. The conversations don't have to take control of the entire meal or be drawn out to be effective—what matters and counts is the re-constitution of the family at mealtime!

Family Meetings

"My parents suddenly announced that we were now going to have family meetings. Great! We never met as a family to discuss anything and I am not excited about this at all. What a waste of time! I could be playing with my electronics rather than sitting around and just listening. Mom said I had no choice."

Contrary to the above example, family meetings can be a wonderful routine to add to your family's bag of healthy tricks. These meetings need to be held weekly and should be a positive experience rather than being structured as a gripe session. Family meetings have been popular for decades and can be used as a family forum for discussion as well as an opportunity for the family to have fun. Setting up a meeting is simple.

The concept of family meetings has been around for decades. It was in the mid 1970s that both of us became acquainted with them. The concept seemed intriguing. Family meetings were an opportunity for families to make time to work on issues and to highlight that collaboration was critical! For the meetings to work, they also needed to incorporate some fun, so all the members would be committed to being involved. Although every family could put its own imprint on the meeting, there are several steps that you could consider in developing a family meeting in your own home. The following list will briefly go over some of the steps and get us to think about how we can put them in our own family:

1. Make a commitment: All beginnings start with an openness to try.

2. Meet at a regular time: This is probably one of the most important aspects of a family meeting; it's planned and we have it at a regular time, preferably once a week, so that the youngsters realize that this is going to occur. The family meeting should be about half an hour to an hour. The meeting could last longer, especially if we add some recreation and fun to end the meeting.

3. How do we start? When first establishing the family meetings, we need to assemble our family and explain why we're doing this. An open conversation could be conducted focusing on the importance of wanting to improve family functioning and relationships.

Once the concept has been agreed upon, we should talk about the jobs that should be filled for the weekly family meetings. Depending on the size of the family, many roles can be formulated and rotated weekly. The leader or the meeting's facilitator is probably the most important role. It is that person who will run the meeting. In the case of a younger child, a parent can help support the youngster. The scribe could be the person who takes notes, the guardian of the agenda can be the person who makes sure that the agenda is completed for the week, and finally one member of the family could be the recreation programmer whose role would be to plan out the fun portion of the evening. That individual could collaborate with their family members and come up with some creative ideas that may include snacks, recreation, games, and perhaps even movies.

4. Make a list of topics: Once the regular format of the family meeting comes up, the guardian of the agenda can make sure that topics for the weekly meeting are collected. The guardian could put on the fridge or on a bulletin board a sheet where members could add subjects for the meeting. For families who have young children who can't write, they can ask an older sibling or a parent to add to the list. Making a list is very important so that an agenda can be made.

5. Leader's role: Make sure that the leader/facilitator is aware of what the agenda is going to be. Attention needs to be given to help each family member feel comfortable being a leader. Early on, parents can help model what a leader does and teach children some of the basic steps (such as how to discuss each item on the agenda). It's important that the agenda is thought about a little bit and clarified, so that when we go through the meeting, it's clear what is expected during the meeting. Planning to get that meeting started and having the leader review the agenda beforehand will be helpful for a seamless meeting to occur. Time for each agenda item should be considered to assess how long topics will have on the agenda.

6. The meeting: To start the meeting, we think that it's really important to institute some kind of ritual. It could be a favorite song that the family enjoys singing. It could be giving compliments to everyone around the circle. In this case, everyone goes around the room and says something good

about what happened to them during the week. This way, we are assured that the meeting starts off in a positive manner.

One ritual that could be discussed in the opening minutes of the meeting is what went well in the family during a specific week and what were some of the challenges. When challenges are discussed it is imperative that the discussions stay focused and don't derail. The mission of the meetings should be to stay civil and on track. This would be a good opportunity for families to practice some of the conflict resolution strategies discussed in the previous chapter.

During the meetings it is important that everyone has an opportunity to talk and express themselves. One potential role of the leader (or perhaps the parent helping the leader) is to identify some family members that perhaps aren't talking as much and to encourage them to engage. Various communication strategies that were identified in a previous chapter will come in handy during this segment of the meeting.

During a portion of the meeting various topics should be discussed as they pertain to the family's functioning. Topics may include how chores are distributed as well as concerns by either parents or children about them. Attention may be given to a specific family problem or future family events. During the meeting, we could also be planning family vacations. Time will need to be designated to get ideas heard and agreements made.

7. Taking notes: Having some type of record of the meeting is valuable. Perhaps you could have the secretary take notes or keep a digital recording of the meeting. Notes are really important because then we will have a record of what was agreed upon and what needs further discussion. The goal of family meetings should be to end in harmony. And that's where we take time for fun. The fun part of the meeting is probably the part that many families cherish.

For example, in our family, our family meetings always ended with some fun games such as playing Ping-Pong, dome hockey, or table games accompanied by a scrumptious dessert that we made beforehand. We have to respect families' other obligations and realize that there may be competing time conflicts. We need to try to get this to become a commitment that goes on over the years. Even when we have teenagers, we need to help them understand that we want them to prioritize our meetings. This may mean that we occasionally need to re-accommodate some of the meetings so they will stay involved. Ultimately, the purpose of a family meeting is the opportunity for the family to work out some differences and learn that family members play an equal and important part in the discussions. Table 1 may be helpful to you as you plan your upcoming family meeting.

Table 1
Family Meeting Planning Sheet

Where will you have the family meeting? Have the meeting away from the setting where the problems occur. Find a **neutral** relaxing environment that does not trigger negative feelings.	
What are the rules for the family meeting?	
How will you set the tone of the meeting? Make the meeting fun. Start with a game or activity that everyone will enjoy.	
What are potential problems you anticipate having in a family meeting?	
What will you do to address the potential problems listed above?	
What has your child done well? Start with a list of the positive accomplishments of your child. Remember to include your child's input in solving problems.	
Which topic will you address first? Always start with the easiest problem to solve first with the goal of establishing the process for solving problems through the family meeting.	

Before ending our discussion on Family Meetings, let's return to the boy that was resistant and hear his new thoughts about family meetings. *"Boy the meeting wasn't bad at all. When it started, Mom had us singing a new family cheer. She was so funny that I laughed and joined in. When we started to talk about a few family things, I felt like talking. Before I knew it, I was telling them everything they wanted to know. In fact, they took some of my suggestions and actually praised me for my good ideas. We ended the meeting playing charades and having ice cream. These meetings aren't so bad. I wonder what we will do next week. Maybe pizza?"*

Sibling Rivalry

"I do not want to share my parents' attention. I still want to be master of my world and I don't want to share it with anyone else. My brother started life getting everything he wanted and needed. Watching my brother reminded me of how it had been when I was King. I do not want to be dethroned."

Sibling rivalry is as old as Cain and Abel, and when we are stuck within the storm, we feel just as old. It is important to realize that siblings have always fought and always will. Conflicts will always arise. Fighting doesn't mean our children don't love each other, but it typically means that they have to learn how to co-exist. If you expect complete peace and harmony between siblings, you're setting yourself up for frustration and disappointment. Fortunately, in the vast majority of instances, the conflict between siblings is nowhere near as serious as the Old Testament example. That is not to say that there aren't serious sibling rivalries that are significantly more dysfunctional. Those circumstances may need more guidance than the suggestions we provide in this section.

Although there are no guarantees, sibling rivalry characteristically is a commonplace occurrence even in the most peaceful of families. While sibling rivalry can be distressing for all members of the family, in general it is perfectly normal. Theoretically, the squabbles help children learn how to be active, positive participants in a close relationship that hopefully continues to be an important bond throughout life.

This can, in part, be attributed to the fact that sibling relationships are often the first significant peer relationships in a child's life. In theory, through these interactions with their siblings, children learn the give and take in relationships and how they like to be treated, and what happens when they treat others in a certain way. Therefore, it is easy to see how this microcosm of human interaction can engender conflict. Sibling relationships, as well as other familial relationships, teach us how to interact and form relationships with others. Sometimes these interactions are influenced by jealousy or a perception of unfairness. We need to do what we can in order to avoid such misrepresentations. They only add fuel to a potential fire.

Conflicts between siblings are also teachable moments for parents, moments in which they can guide and support this unique relationship. Sibling relationships are constantly growing and changing and are much more complex than can be explained by a simple biological predisposition, such as birth order or being predestined to argue, or simply because you have a sibling.

Over the years, we've often heard about arguments and squabbles between siblings. Unfortunately, these squabbles will occur and we will not be able to control them all. However, we have the ability and the opportunity to teach our children how to work out their differences for themselves. Parents should expect the conflicts and have realistic expectations; however, not addressing apparent and even overt sibling conflict prevents future positive sibling relationships.

All families who have more than one youngster recognize that it's difficult for children to work out their own arguments at times. Sometimes, especially with younger children, they may need someone to teach them how to resolve their conflict. We will discuss this position in more detail a little later. However, it behooves parents to act as mentors to teach their children to be effective problem-solvers, rather than be put into the role as both the judge and jury. We can't control all of the battles, but for sure we don't have to get stuck in them. Perhaps the strongest suggestion we can give you is to not get involved with a verdict unless you really have evidence. If you didn't witness or hear anything, it really is unfair to take sides. Avoid these situations at all costs and don't favor one child over the other. Also don't withhold affection to any of your children because of their squabbles. That may make things even worse.

As parents, our job should be to try to teach our children how to resolve their differences without resorting to violence. If we start picking sides or trying to resolve issues without truly understanding what occurred, it could make things worse. Perhaps the most crucial question that is always asked isn't really, "Why do my children fight and argue?" but, "Are there things that can be done that can help me prevent the rivalry from becoming more significant?". We have a couple of suggestions to offer.

Although rivalry is common, Davis and Keyser (1997) assert that many of our reactions to fighting between siblings are based on our perspective. (Such a casual and detached attitude by parents to sibling fighting also serves as an unintended lesson we parents present to our children regarding the role of the parents.) If we maintain a perspective that children are just destined to fight periodically, we will react accordingly. If we feel that children are using the safe sibling relationship in which to explore and practice interactions and expressing emotions, this gives us another way to approach and work with our kids who are having a conflict. Davis and Keyser (1997) concluded that supporting our children with their conflicts with each other is an investment in a family's future. By helping our children in their relationships with their siblings, they can learn the rules of co-existing. These rules will hopefully generalize to their interactions with others.

Strategies to Reduce Conflict with Siblings

As parents, we often can find ourselves in situations where we don't always model the best behaviors that show resolution. Throughout this entire book we've discussed the importance of modeling positive, respectful behaviors, and in doing so, hopefully our children will learn from that. Nevertheless, even when we do all of these positive things, it's very likely that over time our children will have arguments. We need to praise them when they avoid conflicts, but we also need to try to help them learn how to solve unpleasant encounters maturely on their own. We need to be persistent and consistent with our honest praise if they try to work things out on their own. We should also not make one sibling feel inferior and suggest he/she needs to behave like the other one. (You may find this is a common issue with siblings who attend the same schools. Teachers inadvertently may compare siblings, causing one to feel inadequate and inferior.) This form of guilt tripping could make the sibling divide even larger. Faber and Mazlish (1998), in their book *Siblings Without Rivalry*, suggest several ideas to reduce rivalries. The idea of taking the time to listen to our children and hearing their point of view is extremely valuable. Sometimes all children need is a level-headed person to listen to them and help them calm down. We could even brainstorm with them some alternatives of how to de-escalate the problem and possibly resolve it. There are many dimensions in the problem-solving process that should be considered. Utilizing reflective listening skills (discussed in the teen chapter) will help acknowledge to our children that we are trying to listen. We need to help them solve the problems with a respectful tone and attack the problem, not each other. By helping them learn the skills of empathy and reflection, we can show them that we have faith in their ability to resolve their own problems.

In fact, helping our children with problem-solving strategies should be a priority for us. We can help our youngsters become aware of their escalated behavior by showing them how to use a calm voice and monitor if they are in control or not. We can even help by showing them how to stay in control. For example, one idea we often suggest is to help our children learn how to regulate their *temper*-a-ture. If their *temper*-a-ture is high, that may mean they are feeling out of control or very angry. Just like a thermostat, they must learn to adjust their *temper*-a-ture to a comfortable climate. Learning how to cool down may help them to avoid getting into as much trouble. To help with younger children, we can make a large thermometer for them to visualize their anger level and how to maintain control of their emotions. Just knowing they need to cool down before they boil over may be enough to prevent future escalations.

Another useful alternative could be to help our children learn how to filter their anger or discouragement towards their sibling into other more acceptable outlets. For example, they could have their own private journal or drawing book where they can express and release their resentment or feelings in a more desirable manner. We also should encourage our youngsters to be cautious with their words and to not resort to physical reactions. Our children need to appreciate the lasting effects of ill-chosen words uttered in a highly heated and emotional engagement. But above all, they need to be told that physical altercations are not acceptable. Learning how to walk away and not get baited are two other skills that we should talk to our children about. Just like a fish in the water, they need to learn to not take the bait and be drawn into a fight; that way they won't get "hooked."

When interacting with children in a family, it's important for each parent to have time with each individual child and not always spend time with the whole family unit. Individual time gives kids an opportunity to feel that they receive their own specialized attention. While interacting with one of your children, make sure you don't find yourself talking about the other, as this would prove counterproductive. Spending individual time is an idea we strongly endorse because it helps each child feel special. During my children's younger years, we had special days every week where we spent individual time together. These days created memories we cherish. It also behooves parents to encourage their children to have their own friends so they have outlets outside the home. In an upcoming chapter we will discuss friendships in more detail.

Since families may span various years, it's important to look realistically at the constellation and recognize that our youngsters may lack the maturity to solve their own problems. This is very evident with preschoolers who may have conflict several times throughout the day, or even within an hour. When those children are surrounded by their siblings that may be school aged or tweens, the older children may not have patience for them. School-aged children tend to be a little bit bossier, and that's where we also may see some more difficulties. As noted earlier, although we encourage siblings to work things out as much as possible on their own, school-aged children may benefit from our input and direction.

Again, families are living units and we need to know how to function accordingly. Years ago, when working in an urban inner city environment, I worked with children who were constantly bickering and arguing. One day when I came in, the arguing was already going on. In desperation to get their attention, I said in a very stern and loud voice, "Everybody look at your hands." To my surprise I had fifteen boys staring at me wondering why this odd request was given. I quickly followed the first request by asking the group, "If I cut away your palm, what could you do with your fingers?" It was at that moment that many of the children looked in a state of puzzlement. I really wondered if the boys thought I had lost it, and I was about to explode. Eventually, one boy looked up and responded to my question, "You cannot do anything with the fingers because they aren't connected," he retorted. It was at that moment the lights went on for many of the boys. We began to discuss as a group the importance of working together. Just like a palm unites the hand, a group or a family unites various individuals. It is the group, or in our case the family, that unites and connects us all. It's important that we spend the time with our families and teach our youngsters that we need to work hard on becoming united. A united family will be more respectful of individual boundaries and work more closely with each other.

Finally, although we need to work on family unity, there are times that togetherness may not always work. Sometimes siblings and, for that matter, parents need a break from each other. We should consider dividing and conquering our families. It's helpful at times to have respite from the entire family and to divide up while doing things. Dividing and conquering allows us to enjoy the time with a smaller portion of our family and possibly avoid some of the pitfalls of the larger group. Dividing allows parents to realize it is okay to spend time alone with a portion of the family. Sometimes having a break can be refreshing.

Rules for Managing Difficult Conversations and Conflict

All families have conflict from time to time and must learn strategies to resolve the conflict in positive ways. Typically, most arguments when left to fester too long normally only get louder and become more difficult to subdue. As parents, we may begin feeling frustrated and compelled to solve the conflicts utilizing approaches that we may regret. Over reactivity predictably only worsens situations rather than strengthening resolutions. That is why our family needs to have guidelines for handling conflicts. It's like having an extinguisher ready to snuff out a potential fire. Fran Schmidt and Alice Friedman provide one dynamic alternative to consider when conflict arises. They developed a program called *Creative Conflict Solving for Kids*. Within the program, there is one exercise called **rules for fair fighting**. Over the years, we have used some of these rules as a springboard to help all families in dealing with conflict. These rules can be guidelines for any family to employ a civil and constructive conversation among its members. There are five rules of fair fighting. All of the rules could be adapted to suit any family. These are the modifications that we often employ. We suggest four major guidelines:

- *We identify the problem*
- *We attack the problem not the person*
- *We listen to each other*
- *We are responsible for what we say*

All of these rules can be used in any conflict, including differences that need to be settled by siblings. As parents, we should help our children initially clarify the problem that is being confronted and perhaps identify some of the reasons why it has occurred. Parents are encouraged to help their children stay focused on the pressing problem and not become sidetracked with other issues. Unfortunately, too often constructive conversations are derailed because they are sidetracked. This would be similar to following the smoke rather than focusing on the fire. You are always told to put the fire out first! In this case stay with the fire and get it under control before going on to solving other battles.

The second rule is the healthy backbone of the whole exercise. We have to teach our children (and ourselves) to be respectful of all members in the conversation (even when angry) and to attack the problem and not the other person. Often when disruptions occur, many resort to this tactic and it typically is counterproductive! The process only detracts from problem resolution. It usually has negative ramifications, and the problem just gets worse. Teaching children to attack the problem is a valuable lesson. We don't have to criticize each other to solve the issue!

To assist in clarifying these boundaries, Schmidt and Friedman have designated certain behaviors that cannot occur if we are all trying to fight fairly. They call these negative alternatives fouls. Fouls are unacceptable options that cannot be implemented to solve problems constructively. These behaviors include blaming others, threatening, using put-downs, making excuses, and using any form of physical violence. In essence, we're teaching our children (as well as ourselves) that if we are to engage in problem resolution we are going to apply pro-social alternatives.

The third rule follows quite nicely and encourages our commitment to listening to each other. Listening includes respecting each other's boundaries and recognizing that when one person is talking, the other should not interrupt. Ultimately, we learn to listen to each other and apply all of the strategies of reflective and congruent listening that were discussed in the previous chapter. Finally, we need to take responsibility for our words and actions and accept our role in supporting a healthy climate for resolution. There are many other ideas that can be employed for conflict resolution, but fair fighting guidelines are a safe bet as a starting point.

Final Thoughts

Joyce Brothers once said, "When you look at your life, the greatest happinesses are family happinesses." Simply noted, family is the place where you can create memories. Although happiness is our ultimate goal, it doesn't happen by osmosis. We have to work at it, and our efforts shouldn't be at the expense of doing things that matter less. We have to show our children that our family is a priority, and we are willing to put in the time. Throughout this chapter, we have introduced several factors that we all will need to consider to strengthen our family bond. It can be as simple as saying we eat dinners together, and as complex as getting our children to get along. Our efforts will be fruitful when we witness the impact we are making on our family.

Our parting message to you as we end this chapter is that we need to appreciate what is right in front of us, before we lose that window of opportunity. As parents, we need to work on and be committed to making the best of it with our family. Sure, there will be good and bad days and brothers and sisters who don't always get along, but hopefully, the good days will have outnumbered those bad times. Try to spend time focusing on what works for your family and capture those moments while you have them. When you do, those special years will become blessings.

References

Bossard, J. H., & Boll, E. S. (1950). *Ritual in family living: A contemporary study.* Philadelphia, PA: University of Pennsylvania Press.

Davis, L., & Keyser, J. (1997). *Becoming the parent you want to be.* New York: Broadway Books.

Faber, A., & Mazlish, E. (1998). *Siblings without rivalry.* New York: Avon.

Feiler, B. (2013). *The secrets of happy families.* New York: William Morrow

Fulkerson, J., Story, M., Mellin, A., Leffert, N., Neumark-Sztainer, D., & French, S. (2006). Family dinner meal frequency and adolescent development: Relationships with developmental assets and high-risk behaviors. *Journal of Adolescent Health,* 39, 337–345.

Viere, G. (2001). Examining family rituals. *The Family Journal,* 9, 285–288.

CHAPTER 9

The Family That Plays Together Stays Together: Enriching Our Families with Leisure, Sports, and Companion Animals

It seems like yesterday that we competed for the Fine Cup. Several events were incorporated, including tennis, racquetball, Ping-Pong, checkers, and Scrabble. Corey and Sean were on one team. Nya and I were on the other. Each summer on our family vacation, we would divide up into teams and have little competitions (parents versus kids), just for the fun of playing with each other. When the children were younger, Nya used to tell me, "Let's take it easy on them so that they won't get frustrated." As the years went on, it was the boys that had to take it easy on us. They seemed to relish in our defeat. We had to figure out ways to make it easier for us to possibly win. We haven't for quite awhile now, but we continue to smile.

As I look at the Fine Cup, I see various plaques on the trophy commemorating the winners over the years. Although the trophy celebrates the winners, the cup represents a tribute to our family engagement. We laughed and had some great fun during all of these occasions.

For years, families have preached the motto of playing together as a family, and we are firm believers in this. In a world where it seems too easy to not engage, we encourage families to make a point to hang out together and enjoy each other's company. Some of these play times could be designated periods after family meetings, in addition to other days, evenings, or weekends. What is important to the family unit is to make a strong commitment to spend regular, quality time with one another. When a family is able to play and interact with one another positively, typically they will become more closely knit. There is a wealth of options that you can do with your family. The choices are endless and are dependent on many family variables, including interests, competing schedules, finances, and settings. Table 1 identifies several possible resources and activities that families can try. The only thing your family must bring to the table is an open and spirited mind. If this (family time together) will be a new phenomenon in your home, our suggestion is to start slowly, but don't give up on the idea. Having weekly or even monthly special events will typically lead to creating healthy family interactions and memories. We just need to apply the premise and believe that these activities are done for one reason only—FUN!

Table 1

List of Websites for Recreational Activities for Families

WEBSITE RESOURCE	PURPOSE OF RECOURCE	SUGGESTED ACTIVITIES
3–9 Years: Preschool through Lower Elementary		
1. http://www.parents.com/fun/activities/outdoor/weekend-family-activities/#page=2	1. 20 indoor/outdoor activities to do with your children and family	1. Collect leaves, visit a fire station, volunteer (animal shelter, elderly home), have a treasure hunt, put on a magic show, give children old clothes to play "dress up," go to a minor league game, cook/bake

2. http://fun.familyeducation.com/activities-center/toddlers-preschoolers-K12children.html	2. List of fun activities by category for children, indoor, outdoor, games and puzzles, seasonal, gifts, travel, educational	2. Indoor obstacle course, homemade play dough/clay, science activities, 3 legged race
3. https://familysearch.org/learn/wiki/en/Family_History_Activities_for_Children:_3-11	3. Teach your child about the history of their family	3. Help your child research where their family came from, when they came to the US, information on surname, create photo book of family
4. http://www.kinderart.com/teachers/20activities.shtml	4. Indoor activities to do with your children	4. Puppet show, let child blow bubbles with plate, straw, and bubbles, draw on construction paper and decorate, have child guess the "secret" object by only feeling it, have an indoor picnic, create story by each person saying one line then picking the next person to tell next line
5. http://rainydaymum.co.uk/101-ideas-for-a-rainy-summers-day	5. Rainy day activities so your child isn't saying, "I'm bored, there is nothing to do!"	5. Make a rain catcher to see how much rain falls, make mud pies, sing in the rain, jump in puddles, make a bottle shaker with rice/beans then have a kitchen band, make homemade cards for family members' birthdays/events, make a fort with cushions/pillows, snowball sock fight, hide and seek inside
6. http://www.letsmove.gov/active-families	6. Active families, engaging in physical activity with your family and getting your child into the good habit of exercising	6. Play basketball, soccer, or throw a baseball, walk your child to school, go to the park

10–13 Years: Upper Elementary		
1. http://tweenparenting.about.com/od/activitiesgames-hobbies/a/Enrichment-Activities.htm	1. Activities to help enrich your child's life without breaking the bank	1. Foster a passion/hobby, teach your child to sew/crochet, do science experiments at home, see what the YMCA, church, craft store, library have to offer
2. http://everydaylife.globalpost.com/summer-activities-preteens-6020.html	2. Summer activities so your child is not cooped up inside all summer	2. Summer camp, community service projects, library activities
3. http://www.scholastic.com/parents/resources/article/more-activities/fun-history-activities-preteens	3. Fun history and astronomy activities	3. Explore the world of astronomy, search places using Google Earth, look on NASA website at space program, first landing on moon, Apollo 11 launch and mission, send virtual post card to "Spirit" the rover on Mars
14–18 Years: High School		
1. http://www.kidspot.com.au/Parenting-Teen-Fun-family-activities-to-do-with-teens+6751+751+article.htm	1. Usually "fun" and "family activities" don't go together for teens because they would rather be with friends but here are some examples of things you can do with your teen; do things your teen is interested in to make sure they have fun and would want to do something like that again	1. Consult with your teen about what they want to do; have a few options for them, let them bring a friend, don't bring up school grades, messy rooms, etc., go to: amusement parks, go-karting, laser tag, ice skating, indoor rock climbing, big cities, the beach, camping, movie theater, shopping, cosmetics counter for a makeover

2. http://archive.wired.com/geekdad/	2. Ideas for your teen: show your teen you care and pay attention to them and try these fun activities with them	2. Paintballing, miniature golf, comedy clubs; for boys: plan a videogame tournament, for girls: have a spa/sleepover

Sports and youth

Since we started the discussion on making sure that you make time to play with your sons and daughters, we thought it would be helpful to talk about organized sports and our role as parents in these activities. Over the years, we have gone to several ball fields and hockey rinks and have witnessed parents who are out of control and misjudge the experience. Children don't seem to play pick-up games as much as they used to. They seem to be directed to more formalized sporting events where there are coaches, fans, and spectators. Years ago, I (Aubrey) wrote a book with Michael Sachs called *The Total Sports Experience for Kids*, which explores the importance of allowing our children a healthy opportunity to engage in sporting events without always trying to win our approval and support. Children need to be able to enjoy their leisure time not only to decrease stress, but also to have healthy outlets in their lives. Sports can contribute to our physical and psychological well-being and we need to make this an available option. We both realize that registering for sports can be a significant commitment, especially for families who don't have enough social support. However, alternatives need to be considered so the option will be made available. When I (Aubrey) was a young boy, I wanted to play hockey. We were quite poor and couldn't afford the appropriate equipment. That didn't stop my mother from getting me involved. Before I got my first borrowed hockey shoulder pads, I actually borrowed football shoulder pads from a family friend. Not a perfect fit, but it kept me safe while I was having the time of my life.

Leisure, as a term, originated from the Latin word *licere*, which means "to be permitted." Actually, it was the French who redefined the word and developed the word *loisir*, which directly translates to "free time." Over the decades, we have seen an increase of children becoming more sedentary and playing with their electronics rather than engaging in physical sporting activities. Ultimately, the concern that we have and hope to help other parents recognize is we need to give children the opportunity and the outlets to celebrate their own skills and avocations.

Lessons learned through sports

There are many lessons that can be learned when children play sports. The most critical is having fun and the opportunity to express ourselves. Years ago, a good friend of mine, Jon Scolinas, who was a baseball coach at my university (Cal Poly Pomona University) as well as the pitching coach for the USA Olympic team in 1984, identified many lessons that could be learned through sports. These lessons ranged from learning to cope with failure, to developing a sense of commitment. Ironically, we don't appreciate that when you are engaged in sports, there are many life lessons that can be learned. We need to promote the key lessons that can occur from being a member of a team. Team building can foster within children the notion that they are part of something that is larger than them. Years ago, while coaching a group of young teens playing ice hockey, I demonstrated the strength of being a team member. Using five separate strands of string, I asked several boys to break individual pieces. They smiled eagerly as they simply tore the individual pieces of string. However, when they were twined together, the strands were impossible to break. The team was amazed and used the lessons from the strength found within the twinned strings as their impetus for working together. They became a stronger team as they played in their state playoffs. They began to see themselves as invincible. Learning to be a team and making that a priority not only strengthened the bonds on the field but also became a life lesson.

While playing sports, kids have to learn to handle competition and at times confront defeat. These are normal outcomes of playing any sport. How many of us remember a time when we participated in a sport and the outcome wasn't what we wanted? We may have struck out; we may have let in a winning goal. Yet we learned that life didn't stop and it moved on. We believe that kids have the right to learn these lessons from playing, and as parents we do not need to always protect our children from this outcome. Failure is only an event, and does not define the person. We can all learn from defeat.

Sports can also build class and character, especially if those that lead the activities have that objective in mind. The greatest lesson that can be derived from playing on teams is that learning the word *we* is much more important than the word *I*. Remember the old saying, "There is no 'I' in team." Having coaches that truly follow this premise may make your children's sporting years more meaningful, especially if the goals are true to their words.

When we assess the many reasons why children play sports in school and in their recreational time, some people always see it as an opportunity to achieve other aspirations. However, we would disagree. Even when you talk to professional athletes, they would admit that the key to playing sports has to be fun. You have to enjoy the experience to want to participate. Fun must be the pinnacle goal, but playing sports also brings along many other benefits, including improving on your skills. For example, you may not be an elite athlete, but if you can improve your abilities and become better at what you do, that is an accomplishment. Staying in shape and having a chance to exercise are also tremendous benefits. Children need exercise to get away from their sedentary lifestyles. Unfortunately, we see so many children losing interest in sports. Perhaps one of the reasons is that they feel too much pressure from their parents and their coaches. Furthermore as they age, there are new demands on their time. We need to consider ourselves guests in youngsters' sporting lives and not take them over. Parents should avoid living vicariously through their children. It's not our game but our youngsters' opportunities.

Children really need allies when they play, and for that reason we need to be supportive as parents. So many children want their parents to come and watch and possibly assist; however, we believe that it's important for parents to not take over and act irresponsibly. Parents must maintain the perspective that parents are "supportive" allies, not "participants."

Over the years, I've gone to hockey rinks, baseball fields, soccer fields, and football fields and have watched parents behave extremely irrationally as they lose their tempers, get frustrated about why their child isn't playing enough, or feeling the coach is being too hard on their youngster. We also see some parents become overreactive at the events. This can range from yelling and screaming to putting too much pressure on their child. Our question would be: Is this helpful to the child? We all know the answer is no. The behavior typically embarrasses and frustrates the child and makes things worse. If we could be honest and accept this one premise, we think your children would get the most out of playing in organized sports. Recognize that we need to see ourselves as guests in our children's sporting events. That's not to say that we accept this comment literally, but act as proper guests. Remember, we are there to be supportive. It's their game and not ours.

At the end of the day, we need to accept the position that children should be involved for the fun of it. I look at my own boys who both played ice hockey for so many years. I always looked at it as being an enjoyable experience for the family. It wasn't going to be a vacuum of stress and pressure. I think it was for that reason that the boys continued playing throughout their high school years. They enjoyed being there and felt that as parents we were supportive of them, not reactive. Too many parents take the long ride home and criticize or critique everything that their child does. Again, when you put sports into perspective, there are many other benefits that can follow.

The Baskin-Robbins perspective

How do you know when your child is ready to participate in a more competitive level, versus a more relaxed and cooperative level of engagement? This is an important question to consider when selecting the correct level for competition. Some children are more capable of being in a sport that requires more competition while others seem more comfortable in an informal, less competitive option. No one option is better than the other. The only thing that counts is that you select the best choice for the youngster. In the book called *The Total Sports Experience for Kids*, both Michael Sachs and I discuss how the sporting spectrum of options in sports is similar to the numerous ice cream choices of Baskin-Robbins. There are many different kinds of sports and many different levels of competition that a child can participate in; we just need to select the best option for that child. Developmentally, we need to understand that children may be more ready for playing specific sports than others primarily because of their developmental skills. Each of the ages has specific needs that should be considered. Table 2 identifies some of the basic developmental expectations of various sports years.

Table 2
Developmental Expectations of Various Sports Years: A Fact Sheet

	Preschool Age Children	School Age Children	Adolescents
Motor	During the early years, large muscles and basic motor skills develop quite rapidly. Preschoolers increase in their coordination and balance, and their energy level is quite high, especially for short periods of time.	During this age, children's balance and coordination develops and their attention span increases. Their eye-hand coordination is also enhanced during this era. Agility is much more dynamic than it was before in the earlier years.	During the adolescent years, there is improvement in all areas of motor development and coordination. These are young people that can really play sports very well.

Emotional	The preschool child attempts to become more assertive and independent during this time. Children try to exercise more initiative. The child by the age of five or six believes that rules about how to play are absolute and cannot be changed. Therefore, they are much more rigid in playing sports. Friendships are very important and should be considered when coaching these youngsters.	Friendship is crucial during this age period. The child becomes much more aware of other children's feelings. For some children they may have experienced failures and are impacted by them. The competitive spirit seems to develop during this age. They need to practice their skills to improve.	By the late teens, these young individuals should be capable of making better moral decisions. The competitive spirit may increase considerably. Friendships are very important and provide strong psychological support. Teens may choose to opt out of the sporting years because of other competing interests, including spending time with friends, interest in driving, dating, and occupation opportunities.
Implications	Preschoolers should be playing more cooperative sports rather than competitive. They're learning how to play more effectively with others, and that should be the ultimate goal.		The sporting years can be very important for young people beyond just the sports field, but also to keep them in situations that could have positive outcomes.

In addition to the developmental expectations, there are several other variables that should be considered when evaluating if a sport is right for your child, including the level of competition. One is inventorying opportunities and what types of options are available. Depending on where you live, there may be more/less recreational alternatives to engage in. You need to know what type of sport a child is interested in and then begin to make other considerations. You could talk to your child as well as expose him or her to the various options. Once the sport is somewhat selected, you should look at your child's strengths and assets and begin to select what level is best suited. For example, does the child have the capacity to handle more competition, or does the child need more cooperative options so that he or she fits in a bit easier? We also need to look at the accessibility to the activities. Accessibility encompasses topics such as how far of a drive it is to the activity, what kind of time commitment is required as well as the costs and required equipment. It really is important for parents to recognize, although their children want to play, that they need to be involved in the decision-making. Can a parent commit to get the child to all the activities and practices? We think once you commit to the process, you need to do what you can to make sure that the child gets to participate in the activity. This may also help your child realize that commitment applies to the entire family.

Our children do not necessarily view competition in the same way we do, but they quickly learn about winners and losers. The word "competition" in its Latin roots consists of, *com*, which means "with," and *patere,* which means "to seek." The term "competition" actually traditionally means "to seek excellence together." Unfortunately, for some children excellence means being the best. Excellence does not require that you win all your competitive games. Excellence is doing the best you can and learning how to evaluate your performance realistically.

Some leagues that your children will be involved in will emphasize more of a cooperative model. These leagues aren't better or worse, they are just different. The goal of the cooperative leagues is primarily to have the child play with few pressures. The primary goal is fun. The children are taught the fundamentals, but the purpose of the league isn't to develop the child to be the next Mike Trout, at least not at that moment.

On the other hand, more competitive sports take into account not only a child's developmental age and skills, but also his or her ability to handle pressure. As we age, more sporting options become competitive in nature, unless we join an intramural type of league. Strongly competitive leagues may bring a change of focus to the experience. Also, the coaching style may be different. Typically, coaches expect more from the youngsters and may put more pressure on them. That's not to say that the pressure is bad, but we need to make sure our child is ready for this.

At all levels of sports parents need to be vigilant and evaluate the experiences they are providing. Playing in sports should go beyond the actual game. It is about friendship and camaraderie. It's also about making the choices of how much you want to play and how far along you want to go. In essence, we have a lot of things to consider when we register our child, but also as we evaluate the meaningfulness of the experience for them on an ongoing basis. At the end of the day, if we properly help our youngsters navigate through their sporting activities, we'll be able to look back at those memories in a positive way. We'll remember the activities that they participated in, both good and bad. But hopefully, with the proper guidance, good support, and strong coaching, their years of participating in both organized and informal sports will leave them with wonderful memories. All children deserve the opportunity to participate in sports. It's up to us to help figure out how to get them the best opportunity possible.

The Role of Animals in the Family

Animals bless our homes. Their presence enriches our families and warms our hearts. For some families, they bring more meaning into our homes. We all have our stories about our beloved pets. They stood with us in times of great despair, and were our constant companions to play with and talk to. I (Aubrey) have witnessed the significance they have had on my boys and the family as a whole. They have been my boys' confidants, friends, and playmates. In *Our Faithful Companions*, which was published in 2014, I discuss why we are so intrigued with animals and how valuable they are in families with children. While each family functions differently, companion animals impact members within each distinct family in unique ways. More than 150 million households in the United States have at least one pet. That means that six of every ten people in this country have at least one companion animal. According to a 2012 article and a national pet owners survey, families spend about $51 billion annually on their pet's supplies, equipment, and care. Families with young children make up about 60 percent of pet owners in this country and feel that having a pet is healthy for their child, as the pet teaches them responsibility and also enhances their empathy and kindness. Research has demonstrated over and over again that simply having contact with a calm dog or cat can lower blood pressure and anxiety, thus proving that there are real health benefits in ownership. In fact, Dr. Ni (2012) on a blog sponsored by Dr. Oz reported that a Wilkes University study found that stroking a dog for eighteen minutes caused a significant increase in secretory immunoglobulin A (IgA), your body's natural antibody against invading germs. A great deal of research has been generated over the past forty years that explains what many of us have believed for years: having a pet is good for your soul and your health.

Often kids will share that their dog or cat sleeps with them at night and makes them feel safe. Children in single parent households will often feel safer and more secure knowing the dog will alert them to an intruder, serve as a friend, and keep them company when they are alone. Animals may also act as an emotional buffer during stressful situations for children. Many people often comment that they perceive that their dogs or cats are wonderful listeners. Dogs have been domesticated to be excellent responders to our non-verbal communication.

How many of you remember your childhood pets? Did any of you turn to them when you were having a terrible time? Perhaps it could have been a traumatic event in your home or a friend treating you poorly. You often would lie next to your beloved pet and open up your heart. They in turn would possibly nuzzle next to you and non-verbally make you feel better. The affection received from our companion animal while feeling stressed is extremely valuable. The animal brings a sense of stability and offers the comfort we are searching for. For example, my colleague Gail Melson noted in an interview that 75 percent of 10–14 year olds in Michigan preferred to sit by their pets when they were upset, as well as 42 percent of five-year-olds turned to their pet when they are experiencing emotional distress. Finally, it's not uncommon for families to take their pets along on family vacations. We have done this for years, sometimes more successfully than others. Can you imagine a carload filled with two boys, dogs, and a cockatoo all on their way to a log cabin? There was more than singing that could be heard in that minivan so many years ago. Those were wonderful days!

Companionship and friendship are critical in childhood and crucial components to our growth. It makes sense, because the pets take on the roles of being playmates and surrogate siblings. With the changes that we are witnessing in family structure, animals in the home may be providing needed consistency and social support. Pet owners often report feeling closest to their pets, with 85 percent considering their animals as family members.

Probably one of the most enjoyable holidays that my children always loved was Halloween. In *Our Faithful Companions,* I describe a Halloween that was unforgettable. The following is a brief glimpse from the story. "I always smile when I think back to those days, when the boys would sleep with their candies because they worried that I would steal some of them. They knew me pretty well. In fact, I probably would have taken many of the small Snickers bars and candies, if they had left them unguarded. My most memorable of the Halloweens was the time when the family was joined by our oldest dog, Puppy. We all wore costumes and went trick or treating. Sean was Dick Tracy, and Corey was He-Man. Several friends joined our Halloween pilgrimage, but probably the most comical was our dog Puppy, who joined us for the first time. We dressed Puppy as a reindeer. She had a sign on her that said, "I'm a reindeer. I don't speak human. Trick or treat. Can I get some treats, please?" At first she didn't seem very eager to be led around the neighborhood, but quickly as she was rewarded with treats at the doors of various neighbors, her interest was definitely piqued. I will never forget one person who gave her a doggy Popsicle. This thrilled her to no end. Of course, we stopped for a couple of minutes as she devoured her treat. For the next thirty-five to forty minutes, Puppy was first to appear at every door. She sat attentively as she waited for her treat to go into a bucket. Halloween would never be the same again for the boys. To this day, we still smile as we reflect on that day." (p.62)

How to select a pet for your home

There are several questions that families should consider before adopting a pet. You should never make these decisions without thinking them through. Pets are a huge commitment of time, money, and love. A healthy discussion needs to occur before getting the pet, so many of the concerns of pet ownership are discussed and focused. Preparation starts with a conversation of trying to get a grasp of knowing what you are getting into before you actually get a pet.

When selecting a pet for the family, what should be the major variables to consider? They can range from how to select the best pet, to how we make sure that the whole family will be involved in taking care of our new family member. Often, parents assume that they will get their children involved, but what ends up happening is it becomes an added chore for them.

Setting up a schedule and keeping the kids engaged in the care plan of the pet is critical. It is important to remind kids that pets are living beings that have needs. They are completely reliant on us for many of their necessities. In the vast majority of situations, parents can expect a honeymoon phase where the child is completely infatuated with the pet for a period of weeks or even months, but it is completely natural and normal for some children to outgrow their interest. That is when we need to help them make responsible choices. Having a healthy and happy dog or cat can be achieved through multiple caregivers in the family who all are willing to pitch in. We just need to make sure that we organize the care plan. We need to be patient and set realistic expectations. Fighting about your plan is not healthy for your relationship with your children, and it will also not benefit the pet.

If you are considering adding a pet to your family, there are many suggestions that we can give you. Dr. Stanley Coren, Professor Emeritus at the University of British Columbia, suggests that the most important variable to consider when selecting a companion animal (particularly a dog) is the size and the activity level of the species. In an interview that was originally published in *Our Faithful Companions*, Coren suggests that smaller and less active dogs seem to relate well with people who were not very active. Families should consider matching the physical needs of a dog to their own personal lifestyle. He also believes that an understanding of the characteristics of specific breeds is extremely important in the selection process. You need to realize that even when puppies age, their cognition will be roughly equivalent to that of a two-year-old child. That is not to say that they will always be active, but they will need our attention and supervision. Sometimes we want to spontaneously adopt pets without realizing some of the challenges that will ensue if they are neglected. By preparing ahead, we may even consider waiting a bit until we feel we can do this right! Adoption should be for the lifespan of the pet. We need to be committed for the long run!

On the other hand, Francois Martin Ph.D., a senior leader of the Behavior Group at Nestle Purina, also agreed that it is important to strongly consider your lifestyle before making a selection. Francois suggests that you need to select a potential pet based on the individual animal and his/her temperament. What that means is that you need to take the time to observe the pet you are adopting and try to discern if he/she is the right choice for your family. You should be open-minded and ask many questions while considering what type of pet will be the best fit for your family.

I argue that the first step to pet selection must be that you need to think about how you live your life, rather than considering a specific species/breed of animal. You really need to know yourself before you add another being to the equation. If you are by nature a sedentary person, should you adopt an active breed such as a beagle? Unfortunately, too many people have false expectations of how and what an animal will contribute to their lives. If you don't like exercise, having a pet typically will not change your activity level. As parents, we need to be realistic with how a pet will fit into our family and how we will as a family adjust to having a new member. We both feel pets are crucial, but if you don't have the time to integrate a pet into your family's lifestyle at the moment, it may make sense to wait until you are truly ready.

Knowing your lifestyle also includes what you do on a daily basis as well as on the weekend. For instance, does your family travel a lot? If you do, is it fair to have a companion animal (especially one that you will leave at home often)? How do you deal with your downtime? Are you more sedentary or more active? Do you enjoy going to sporting events, or are you a person who likes being out in the outdoors? What are the ages of your children and are you all willing to make adjustments to your lifestyle to live responsibly with a companion animal? These questions need to all be considered.

You should always try to make an adoption decision away from the animal. Go home and think about it. There really isn't an exact science to matching. Any time you add a new dog to your family, whether a puppy or an adult, purchased from a breeder or adopted from a shelter, there are bound to be a few bumps in the road. However, if the family feels bonded to their pet, they are much more likely to commit to working through any short-term challenges.

To help you with selecting the best pet for your family, I developed the Lifestyle Attributes for Pet Selection (LAPS) in *Our Faithful Companions*. Please consider utilizing the LAPS as you possibly select your next pet for the family. Whatever pets you and your family eventually select or have selected, our hopes are that it will be a blessed union and one that will strengthen not only your family bonds but also your bond with all living beings.

Table 16
Lifestyle Attributes for Pet Selection (LAPS)

Reprinted with permission from Fine A. (2014) *Our Faithful Companions: Exploring the Essence of Our Kinship with Animals.* Crawford CO: Alpine Publications

The following Lifestyle Attributes for Pet Selection (LAPS) survey is a tool I have developed to help you get a better understanding of the specific needs and circumstances of your particular life and family. While the LAPS has not been validated, I believe it can still be helpful to you in understanding the type(s) of companion animals that may be best suited for you and your situation. Make sure you answer honestly, as you are the only one who will ever see this, and the more honest you are, the better you will be able to select which companion animal may be a great fit for you to add to your family!

Time

I work long hours

1	2	3	4	5
Never		Sometimes		Usually

I travel a lot for work or pleasure

1	2	3	4	5
Never		Sometimes		Usually

I have time to exercise my companion animal

5	4	3	2	1
Never		Sometimes		Usually

I have time to train my companion animal

5	4	3	2	1
Never		Sometimes		Usually

I have time to play with my companion animal

5 4 3 2 1
Never Sometimes Usually

I have time to socialize my companion animal

5 4 3 2 1
Never Sometimes Usually

I have other family members who need a lot of time and attention as well

1 2 3 4 5
Never Sometimes Usually

A score greater than 18 indicates that you are a very active person! A companion animal that does not take up as much time such as a cat, rabbit, or rodent may be a better fit for you.

Finances

I can afford all the things needed to first bring my companion animal home

1 2 3 4 5
Never Sometimes Usually

I can afford the routine/preventative care my companion animal would require

1 2 3 4 5
Never Sometimes Usually

I can afford to provide care for my companion animal in an emergency

1 2 3 4 5
Never Sometimes Usually

I can afford day-to-day expenses for my companion animal

1	2	3	4	5
Never		Sometimes		Usually

I can afford to have someone care for my animal if I am away

1	2	3	4	5
Never		Sometimes		Usually

I can afford to care for my animal for several years

1	2	3	4	5
Never		Sometimes		Usually

I can afford the pet deposit my landlord requires

1	2	3	4	5
Never		Sometimes		Usually

A score greater than 18 indicates that you can probably afford an animal that might have more start-up and long-term expenses. Examples of animals that can be more expensive to maintain are dogs, horses, and certain species of birds.

Space

I have a large enough backyard for the companion animal I am considering

5	4	3	2	1
Never		Sometimes		Usually

I have a large indoor living area for the companion animal I am considering

5	4	3	2	1
Never		Sometimes		Usually

I have enough space to contain all of the things my companion animal requires

5	4	3	2	1
Never		Sometimes		Usually

I know my landlord will be okay with my companion animal living with me

5	4	3	2	1
Never		Sometimes		Usually

A score of greater than 11 indicates a smaller animal may be more appropriate for you. You may want to consider a cat, aquarium, or rodent.

Family Considerations

There are people I live with that have allergies to certain animals

1	2	3	4	5
Never		Sometimes		Usually

There are people I live with whose other health concerns need to be considered

1	2	3	4	5
Never		Sometimes		Usually

There are small children or elderly people that live with me

1	2	3	4	5
Never		Sometimes		Usually

There may be small children or elderly people living with me in the future

1	2	3	4	5
Never		Sometimes		Usually

My family is always on the go, or not home very often

1	2	3	4	5
Never		Sometimes		Usually

I have other companion animals in my family that will need to be introduced

1	2	3	4	5
Never		Sometimes		Usually

A score greater than 15 indicates that you have many people in your life who will need to be considered when adding a new companion animal to the family. You may want to research hypoallergenic animals, or if there are any animals not recommended for people with certain health conditions. Dogs, cats, and rodents can make great companion animals for the children and the elderly, but size and energy need to be taken into account.

Pet Care

I have enough time to contribute to care for this companion animal

5	4	3	2	1
Never		Sometimes		Usually

I will primarily be responsible for looking after this companion animal

5	4	3	2	1
Never		Sometimes		Usually

I have someone who will take care of this companion animal when I am gone

5	4	3	2	1
Never		Sometimes		Usually

I will provide training for this companion animal

5	4	3	2	1
Never		Sometimes		Usually

A score of greater than 11 indicates you do many things with your time. A companion animal that does not require as much constant care may be something for you to consider. Examples of animals that are more content to be alone for long hours include cats, reptiles, amphibians, and fish.

Final Thoughts

When families have reunions, they are often filled with nostalgia of days gone by. The memories are built on our lives of the past and our way of life of the present. Each day, our children go to sleep and wake up one day older. There is nothing magical or mysterious about that! This is a fact of life! Either we make the best of these moments or we miss these windows. We suggest that you hold onto these moments and build upon them. Those families that engage with one another and work on enjoying and respecting each other are families that will leave a legacy for the future.

Thoroughout this chapter, we have made many suggestions to make the dance richer and livelier in your home. The truth is, all of these ideas will take time and effort, but many, including both of us, believe it will make family living more enjoyable. Homes were built for living and hopefully your family will build a home that will invite pleasure. Albert Einstein once stated, "Rejoice with your family in the beautiful land of life!" This simple commentary has direct meaning to all of us. We put the efforts in working with our children so we can enjoy our lives as a family. Perhaps Albert was very correct! Turn on the music, dance, and rejoice with your family while you are all together. It will be time well spent.

References

American Pet Products Association (2011). *American Pet Products Association national pet owners survey.* Greenwich CT: APPA.

Coren, S. (1998). *Why we love the dogs we do: How to find the dog that matches your personality.* New York: Fireside.

Fine, A. & Sachs, M. (1997). *The total sports experience for kids.* South Bend: Diamond Communications, Inc.

Fine, A. H. (2014). *Our faithful companions: Exploring the Essence of Our Kinship with Animals.* Crawford, CO: Alpine Publications.

Martin, F. (personal communication, April 5, 2013).

Melson, G. (2000). Companion animals and the development of children: Implications of the biophilia hypothesis. In A. H. Fine (Ed.) *The Handbook on AAT (1st edition)* (pp. 376–382). San Diego, CA: Academic Press.

Ni, M. (2012, June 7). Live longer with pets [Web log post]. Retrieved from http://www.doctoroz.com/blog/mao-shing-ni-lac-dom-phd/live-longer-pets

CHAPTER 10

Pointing Your Child to a Life of Resiliency: A Lifetime Journey

Fall Seven Times, Stand Up Eight
Japanese Proverb

Early in June of 2014 the world of hockey fans watched the Los Angeles Kings do what many thought was impossible. They became the living comeback kids to win the Stanley Cup. It took them over seven overtime games and four comebacks to reach hockey's Holy Grail and win the Stanley Cup. Twenty-six games were played and 1,670 minutes ticked on the clock for the Kings to turn naysayers into believers. They had what some teams were missing. They believed in themselves and never gave up! Throughout the playoffs, the media kept focusing on the magic ingredient that transformed the team. The word they used was "resilience." This word is frequently described as a mystical elixir that transforms people into believing they are invincible. Our question is: What does it take for our kids to become comeback kids—kids that won't take "no" for an answer and are willing to do what it takes to overcome?

Over the years, we have met many children that we would today call resilient. Resilience allows individuals to adapt to adversity and trauma and to work through their personal challenges. The key to a resilient outcome is the person's ability to bounce back. It's our ability not only to recover from tough experiences but to rebound and make the change that makes the difference.

Wouldn't it be wonderful if we could help all of our children to become comeback kids? We could weatherproof them so they could handle the storms and find hidden rainbows. In education we emphasize the three Rs, which include reading, writing, and arithmetic. The phrase the "three Rs" was initially conceived by Sir William Curtis in the late 1700s because of the strong R sound at the beginning of the three major academic subjects: **Reading**, **wRiting** ("riting"), **aRithmetic** ("rithmetic") (Timbs, 1825). Perhaps the basics should be expanded to include a fourth R: resilience. In this way we would prepare all children to succeed academically and socially; they would also display intenalized skills that will support their perseverance for securing a better life.

So many questions may come to our minds as we think about our own children. Are people born to become more resilient, or is resilience something that grows within us? Why are many people more prone to giving up, while others seem to persevere and move forward? Are we genetically predisposed to be more resilient or are these traits environmentally engrained in us? These are the themes and questions that will be answered in this chapter. We will conclude our presentation by providing you with guidance on how to create a survival backpack with its compass that points your child towards resilience.

Defining Resilience

Simplistically, resilience in childhood can be understood as the ability to keep going during difficult times, whether it is something extremely earth shattering or something mild. We think that most people see resiliency as the ability to bounce back from adversity and to persevere. Ginsburg and Jablow (2006) report in their book, *A Parent's Guide to Building Resilience in Children and Teens*, that resiliency is the capacity to rise above challenging circumstances (p. 4). This process allows people to move forward in life with hope, optimism, and confidence, even in adversity.

In order to become resilient, we first must build and strengthen our response to stress through practice. When we do this, we gradually gain new coping skills and learn to face challenges more specifically. Perry (2006) states that life is full of surprises and challenges for some, distress and trauma for others. Children facing challenging outcomes will show a range of responses. Some will regress in facing even the minor unavoidable stress of a typical day at school. Other children learn to tolerate and will even continue to thrive in the face of significant distress. It's this bounce-back factor that underlies the success that we all seek.

There is a powerful correlation between high self-worth or high self-esteem and resilience. People who feel good about themselves are more often people who will not give up on things. They realize that failures are events that don't reflect their entire being. We can turn these events or mistakes into positive future outcomes.

When talking about resiliency, we can't separate the fact that interpersonal skills, our ability to ask for help and to connect with others, as well as our ability to express ourselves, are all related to positive, healthy flexibility. Kids who are able to talk to and relate with others with confidence feel better about themselves. This usually leads to more possible life outcomes. Resilience also has to do with looking at things realistically. Not everyone is going to be able to run a marathon at an Olympian pace; however, when we evaluate ourselves realistically, we realize it is equally important to finish the races of life we are involved in rather than always winning them. In essence, setting realistic goals is probably a major dimension of resiliency. Being aware of our own weaknesses and strong points allows us to work harder to make changes in our lives. Children with resilience seem to develop their sense of mastery and a belief that their own efforts can make a difference in an outcome. This sense of mastery seems to be a fundamental key promoting change.

What most parents want for their children is for them to be happy and successful in life. A key question that we are often asked is: What can families do to equip their children to persevere? What elements do we put into their backpacks of life that promote the stamina not to give up? As parents our role is to help our children build their inner capabilities so that they can deal with the challenges that the world will throw at them. As we know, children have many obstacles that they have to deal with. Some possible issues include teachers who are critical of their work, friends who choose not to hang out with them, and parents/coaches who don't acknowledge effort and individual differences. Children who have a healthier level of resilience navigate more effectively through all of these challenges and seem to have stronger support systems. Such a child can grow up to have what is needed to be a resilient adult. In the adult years, these will be the individuals that will be able to overcome adversity more easily and move forward.

Throughout this book, we've emphasized that one of the most critical goals in bringing up our children is to raise positively oriented adults who can handle the bumps and bruises that life will offer them. Our dance with our children will take us through numerous roads and areas. Our role needs to be supportive and help lead our children through the complexities of life. We all hope that our children will have blessed lives filled with wonderful outcomes, but we realize that that may not be completely realistic. One of the aspirations that we have as parents is to help prepare our children to cope with difficult and challenging events so that they will be able to bounce back. We also hope that we can teach our children how to recognize happiness when it's right in front of them.

Years ago, Brooks and Goldstein (2001) wrote a book called *Raising Resilient Children, Fostering Strength, Hope, and Optimism in Your Children,* and a comment caught our eye. They noted, "For too long, we have been influenced by a culturally driven deficit thinking model. Consequently, as our children are experiencing increasing problems, our efforts, as parents, have been directed towards how to fix these problems" (p. 290). Like most ailments in our society, we look for quick fixes, rather than rooting out the problem. Instead of always trying to fix the voids in our children's lives, we should also assure them that sometimes things don't always work out the way we planned. We need to equip our youngsters with healthy coping mechanisms so that they can effectively confront problems and work towards a resolution. We can act as role models and provide them with living examples for coping as well as acting as supports and resources for them. Our youth need more models in their lives rather than judges and critics.

It seems so arduous to bring up a child and to give him or her what is needed to become self-sufficient; however, so many children lead their lives self-destructively and often are frustrated with who they are. They are also either overprotected or not protected at all. We need to equip our children with tools that will help them become more connected and self-sufficient if they are to learn to dance more confidently with others. That means we need to make ourselves more available to our children, perhaps doing nothing more than listening and paying close attention to their emotions. These options should be considered as strategies supporting the Parent-Child Dance. By being available to them, we demonstrate their importance in our lives. While playing with them or creating other family rituals and history, we help them see our interest in their lives; hopefully we also acknowledge the good choices they're making. Of course, there always will be children who will struggle and make poor choices sometimes, or a lot of the time. We should continue our efforts and not give up. All children have their own unique treasures within them, but they may be buried underneath self-doubt. Our role in their cases would be to help remove the tarnish and help them polish their treasures. In essence, they will need our continued guidance.

Why Do We Want Our Children to be Resilient?

The question seems rhetorical because in reality, all of us would like to have children who are inoculated to cope and feel happy with their lives. All parents seem to want to raise their children to have an astonishing life rich with experiences. For some, if they had their way, they would want their children to never experience life's misfortunes such as pain of pressure, bullying, divorce, or poverty. Nevertheless, parents cannot protect children from all the negatives of life. I often use the analogy of waving "fairy dust" over children's heads to explain this dilemma. As a magician, we perform miraculous feats, but in reality, our miracles are merely illusions. Like mortal magicians, parents can't help their children avoid all the negatives in life. We need to expend our energies helping them learn how to rise above these negatives. Our role is to equip our children so they can navigate through their challenges in life more successfully. In fact, how will children appreciate what they have if they haven't ever seen or experienced some of these tragedies? Our role is not to have our children avoid all sorrow, but to teach coping strategies and alternative ways of dealing with difficult situations. They must also learn that they can perceive negative events as opportunities for growth rather than personal defeats.

In essence, there is no magic bullet. There is no simple answer to guarantee resilience in every situation. We can only help our children learn to negotiate and work through things. We can help them build their confidence so they will believe they have the power within them to make things work. Building resilience isn't just periodically watering a plant. It is an ongoing practice that's developmental and preventative. It is a process where children will armor themselves and develop internal strengths, including a sense of character.

Years ago, the state of California developed a task force to define self-esteem in the citizens of the state. The outcome was a definition that described self-esteem as a social vaccination. The vaccination inoculates people from life's misfortunes. Those individuals who have healthier self-esteem will be more likely to be more resilient to the tragedies in life that could occur. Resiliency, like healthy self-esteem, is that vaccination that hopefully will give our youngsters the impetus to persevere even in times when things don't go right. Life isn't always that bowl of cherries in fairy tales. Children who develop a healthier level of resiliency eventually will realize that life will be filled with ups and downs. Hopefully, we will weather the downs, and the positive outcomes in our lives will help us appreciate our efforts. Failure is a fact of life, but it should not deter our children from learning how to cope with it and make lemonade out of lemons.

What Are the Signs of a Resilient Child?

It's easy to identify an un-resilient child. These are children who don't seem to have strong coping mechanisms and seem to get befuddled, frustrated, fearful, or angry when things don't seem to work out. They typically have negative self-talk and doubt their capabilities. On the other hand, what are some of the features that stand out in youth who are resilient? Perhaps the most notable characteristic is their ability to bounce back. They are like rubber balls and seem to get right back up. They seem resistant to giving up! Ginsberg (2011) compared bouncing back up to buoyancy. When pushed under water, our bodies instinctively rise up to the surface (p. 4). Children who have resilience seem to rise above their challenges.

The key to resilience is buoyancy—the ability to bounce up and rise back to the surface. When a child is resilient, he/she is able to move on and continue on his/her path, even in times when obstacles are in front of him/her. For example, when Aubrey's elder son, Sean, played hockey as a goalie, he understood that goals were going to be scored. A player was not expected to stop all the shots that were taken on him. He just needed to stop most of them that he realistically could save. Fortunately, there are youngsters that are capable of letting go of a goal that was just scored and are now thinking about how they will save the next one. Being resilient is letting go of things that bring us down, and recognizing that there are still opportunities to attain success. In essence, it means giving ourselves permission to let go of the ones we haven't saved, and appreciating and acknowledging the ones that we have. Resilience has to do with the ability to reframe one's perspective in terms of failure. For example, some children may consider if the failure was entirely the product of their personal shortcomings or if there were other variables that entered into it. These children may learn that they need to leverage their strengths to compensate for their weaknesses. Fundamentally, children who are resilient recognize that all humans fail! No one lives a failure-free life.

Resilience comes from children experiencing success and viewing that success in a reasonable manner. Recognizing that one person's success may not be another person's success is something to consider. As children age, they need to be given reasonable control over their lives. In this manner they can learn to become positive risk-takers. They also can begin to appreciate the need to learn to be responsible for their day. Sometimes they will learn this by us modeling healthy ways of coping.

We need to demonstrate to our children that they are lovable and capable. By doing so, we can demonstrate to them that we believe that they can become even better at what they do and stronger than who they think they are. The important thing is that they learn to stay positive and apply healthy strategies to confront noxious conditions.

Our own private self-talk impacts resiliency. Self-talk gives a glimpse of how we think. Self-talk impacts the way we think. For example, when we use a lot of negative self-talk, such talk contaminates the way we think and typically taints the way we react to situations. The process often weakens our body and leaves us feeling more defenseless. The old saying—"How you think about your concerns will either relieve or aggravate them"—is very true. This thought seems quite apropos to explain the way we think. In essence, resilience impacts a belief system that is built on optimism. Optimists have very different coping mechanisms. People who are optimistic think in positive terms and believe that challenges are surmountable. In short, they are those who see the glass half full rather than half empty. They are individuals who believe that people are capable of change if they choose to act. Perhaps a key to equipping our children to become more resilient is helping them discover that they have the power within themselves to make the change. We now know through documented research that optimism improves our quality of life. Our optimistic thinking promotes our physical health and our ability to combat illnesses. Indeed neurochemistry bears this out. Negative thinking releases various neurotoxins like cortisol that contribute to feelings of depression. Optimistic thinking stimulates happy neurochemicals like serotonin and dopamine that enhance feelings of well-being and confidence. It seems that this healthy way of thinking enhances our immune system to attack adversity. Feeling better about the future may directly help us actually feel better.

In a study reported in the Journal Psychological Sciences (2010) and released in a news release by the Association of Psychological Sciences, Suzanne Segerstrom of the University of Kentucky and Sandra Sephton of the University of Louisville studied how law students' expectations about the future affected their immune response. The study consisted of about 125 first-year law students. The researchers examined the relationship between the students' personal optimism and cell-mediated immunity (CMI). CMI is known to play a central role in protecting people against viral infections. Their results suggest that being more optimistic about outcomes promoted better immunity against some infections.

Viktor Frankl, the noted neurologist and psychiatrist, stated in *Man's Search for Meaning* that everything can be taken from a man but one thing: the last human freedom to choose one's attitude toward, any given set of circumstances. The book stemmed from Dr. Frankl's insights into life after being an inmate in the Nazi concentration camps. He believed we could find meaning in both the good and bad events of life. In so many areas of life the way we think about things is an extremely important approach to coping. Having a sense of optimism or a healthy belief will at times be what is needed to persevere.

Martin Seligman (2006), who is considered the father of positive psychology, writes in his book *Learned Optimism: How to Change Your Mind and Your Life,* "Life inflicts the same setbacks and tragedies on the optimist as the pessimist. But the optimist weathers them better...the optimist bounces back from defeat and picks up and starts again. The pessimist gives up and falls into depression. Because of his resilience, the optimist achieves more at work, at school and on the playing field. The optimist has better physical health and may even live longer" (p. 207). Optimism is the oxygen that breathes resilience into our blood stream. It allows us to overcome tragedies by believing in a silver lining. Winston Churchill once said, "A pessimist sees the difficulty in every opportunity; an optimist sees the opportunity in every difficulty."

Factors Promoting Resilience

In so many ways it's easier to discuss young people who are resilient and explain why that occurs versus youngsters who have challenges with resilience. We struggle with understanding why that occurs. Over the years, there are many variables that people have recognized that support resilience in all beings. Here is a glimpse of some of these factors.

A. Supportive parents

We believe that the presence of at least one unconditionally supportive parent is crucial. As parents, we play a tremendous role in letting our children know that they're okay, even if they're not the best at what they do. Letting them know that we appreciate what they're doing, and how they're doing it, is crucial. According to the American Psychological Association's document *The Road to Resilience*, helping our youngsters develop close family relationships and helping them with their friendships are key elements to being resilient. Having social support is something that helps individuals recognize the importance of being part of a whole community. There are several reasons why social supports are critical to acquiring healthy resilience. It is apparent that having valuable social supports mitigates the stresses that children feel because they're surrounded by people and have other resources that will support them. Research has shown that people who perceive high levels of social support may experience less stress and cope more effectively, even in times of great need. It is evident that perceived social support is an ingredient that promotes resilience.

Children who are more resilient traditionally feel appreciated and loved by others. Additionally, research has shown that having a caregiver who helps soothe and calm down a child may make it easier for the young person to cope. Unfortunately, an anxious and inexperienced parent/caregiver can ultimately shape a child to become more reactive and less capable in dealing with stress. We need to help children realize that they are capable human beings who can change if they're willing to make a change. Applying resilience does relate to internal confidence and a willingness to be open to change at any time.

B. Temperament

It seems that some children are born with a higher threshold for tolerating stress, or distress, and seem to roll with the punches. However, there are some children that are born with a more senstitive temperament. These youngsters seem to have more difficulty coping because they often get their feelings hurt. Children who are easier to comfort are more likely to become resilient later in their lives. There are many things that children can do to promote their internal endurance, but it seems realistic to point out that children's resilience is dependent on both their genetic make-up and what they have learned in life. In essence, you cannot separate the nature and nurture implications.

C. Putting things into perspective

Learning to keep things in perspective is an important trait. Some people become so invested in an outcome that they often don't see the forest for the trees. They are so driven in terms of their expectations that when things don't come to the expected fruition they feel that their world is shattering. This can be a very risky alternative because you can walk away feeling empty and disappointed. Taking time to gain perspective is critical. People who seem to be more resilient seem to put things into a perspective and analyze things with a more objective viewpoint. Having a positive mindset and realizing that the world won't come to an end is a useful trait. It usually allows people to see a silver lining and promotes their willingness to not give up!

D. Taking care of yourself

Simply said, good health supports resilience at any age. Whenever possible, children should be taught and encouraged to eat healthfully and take care of their bodies. A healthy body has been correlated to numerous mental health benefits, including enhanced mood states, decrease in stress, enhanced body image, and enhanced cognitive skills. All of these benefits are living proof that a healthy body often correlates with a healthy mind. We need to help our children find balance in their lives that include a healthy lifestyle. As ancient Buddhism urges, "It is every person's duty to keep his or her body in a state of good health." If good health is not achieved, "we shall not be able to keep our mind strong and clear." Ultimately, helping our children develop more healthy lifestyles will enhance their capacities to become more resilient.

What's Our Role as Parents in Building Resilience?

We cannot be totally responsible for the well-being of our children but we can be instrumental in teaching them how to make their lives easier on a daily basis. As parents, we need to concentrate more of our energies on changing what we can support in our children rather than placing all our energies in trying to the change the world around us (Brooks and Goldstein, 2001). It's important to be realistic in what our roles are and the impact we can have on our child's overall mental health.

Perhaps one of our first missions is to teach our children not only how to succeed but also how to fail. Hopefully, we will be able to instill in our children that failure is an event, not a person. They can learn from failed outcomes and turn them around. Our children also need to learn to be realistic with their skills and realize that they don't always have to be the best to do the best. They just need to learn to do their best and give an honest effort. It seems today that many children believe that they have to be the best at everything they do, rather than accepting their own personal excellence.

Children also have to learn to be risk-takers. Where would we be today without people like the Wright brothers or Gandhi, who were willing to take chances to make a difference in the lives of others? Risk-taking means not being afraid of failing but recognizing that we have the abilities to make a difference. As parents, our role is to help our children become risk-takers and to reach for new achievements. Pope John XXIII accurately reflects our belief about reaching for your dreams with his statement, "Consult not your fears but your hopes and your dreams. Think not about your frustrations, but about your unfulfilled potential. Concern yourself not with what you tried and failed in, but with what it is still possible for you to do."

As parents, it behooves us to support our children's dreams and let them know that goals are reachable. We should also have activities in our home life that gently push our children out of their comfort zone and help build their capacity to deal with stressors. There are so many examples that can be given to illustrate this position. Many years ago, Sean (the eldest son of Aubrey) was going to play a short piece in a piano recital. Although he enjoyed his time playing piano, he was also quite busy with school and hockey and didn't always practice as much as he needed. He wanted to be part of the recital because he respected his teacher. That day turned out to be a great teachable moment for Sean. As he began to play his song, *The Phantom of the Opera,* he very quickly made several mistakes. Rather than falling apart, he decided to stop playing. He looked towards the audience and said quite confidently, "I would like to have a re-do. I didn't have a chance to practice the way I should have, but I wanted to play because it was important to my teacher." Once he was given that next opportunity, he nailed his second try. He was beaming with pride, but perhaps not as much as observed on the faces of his parents and teacher. They were proud that Sean had not given up and gave the performance his best effort.

Being a risk-taker is being willing to recognize that we are not always going to be the best. It also means that we are not afraid of having a few bumpy roads. Just look at the LA Kings. They had many bumps on their pathway to achieving the Stanley Cup, but they didn't let those bumps get in their way of achieving their ultimate goal. We as parents can be helpful by trying to provide our children with life opportunities where they feel challenged, but we believe that these encounters are within their reach to accomplish. When we frame challenges, children begin reasonably to feel more competent attempting opportunities that are a bit more difficult. We can also help our children by modeling for them ways to cope and to handle more challenging situations. We need to help our children appreciate what the boxer Muhammad Ali once stated: "To be a great champion you must believe you are the best. If you're not, pretend you are."

Perhaps an area of resiliency that isn't often discussed is how to teach children how to cope with stress and frustration. Children need to learn how to reduce their stress so that they won't feel overwhelmed. They also need to capture their sense of happiness and a healthy sense of humor. A sense of humor not only makes us happy, but it also can reduce tension in stressful times. Humor allows us to take life less seriously and reduces stress hormones such as cortisol and adrenaline. Patch Adams, the famous physician who identified the therapeutic importance of laughter, once stated, "The most radical act anyone can commit is to be happy." Happiness generates happy thoughts and with those thoughts some self-inflicted roadblocks dissipate.

Raising children has its ups and downs in both good and bad times. We need to be diligent in our roles and try to stay calm. When mistakes are made, we need to help our children understand that they can learn from these blunders and continue forward. Children seem to do best when they feel loved and understood. I (Aubrey) can recall when both of my boys played hockey. I never really cared about the score. After all of their games, I would always consistently ask them how they were doing and if they had fun. The conversations about their performance would only occur when they were willing to discuss it. In essence, we can try to protect our children from harm's way, but we need to realize that in the end the child holds the power for change.

One of the most difficult tasks in helping our children to formulate a resilient mindset is to encourage them to use healthy self-talk even in times of failure. Again, empathy, congruent communication, and showing our children that we appreciate their efforts are critical elements in making our youngsters believe more in themselves. They need allies that are supportive rather than enemies that bring them down.

Finally, we need to promote in our children a sense of self-control. They need to learn to be humble and use that control to attain their achievements. Children need to know that there is a way for them to get to their promised land. They need, however, to have their own hope and an awareness that we believe in them as well.

What to Put into Our Child's Backpack of Resilience

As we have explained, children who are resilient seem more capable of weathering their storms of life. Although we cannot guarantee that all children will become comeback kids, we believe that as parents we can contribute to their successes by promoting certain beliefs. We have often been told that you are what you eat. In the same fashion, we will argue that your ability to become resilient is dependent on many factors that can be influenced. As we prepare our children for their journey for life, it behooves us to make sure that they have what they need in their back pack for a safe and enlightening adventure. Backpacks are perhaps one of the best tools ever invented for hiking. When packed efficiently and organized with what you need, the backpack will help promote stability and comfort in your trip.

The following are the elements that need to be incorporated in our child's backpack of resilience. Although many of these ingredients have been discussed theoretically earlier in this chapter, this section will discuss these essentials in a practical manner. When these elements are properly placed in the backpack and utilized, it is more likely that our child will become more resistant to the negative outcomes that he/she will confront. It is only appropriate that we use the acronym **ARCHERS** to help identify the specific essentials that should be packed. Within this unique backpack, there will be seven arrows pointing your child towards resiliency.

ARCHERS

A- Attitude

R- Responsible for your day

C- The three Cs–*Confidence*, *communication*, and the use of your internal *compass*

H- Happiness, humor, and health

E- Effort

R- Risk-taking

S- Self-appreciation

The Backpack of Resilience: The Essentials

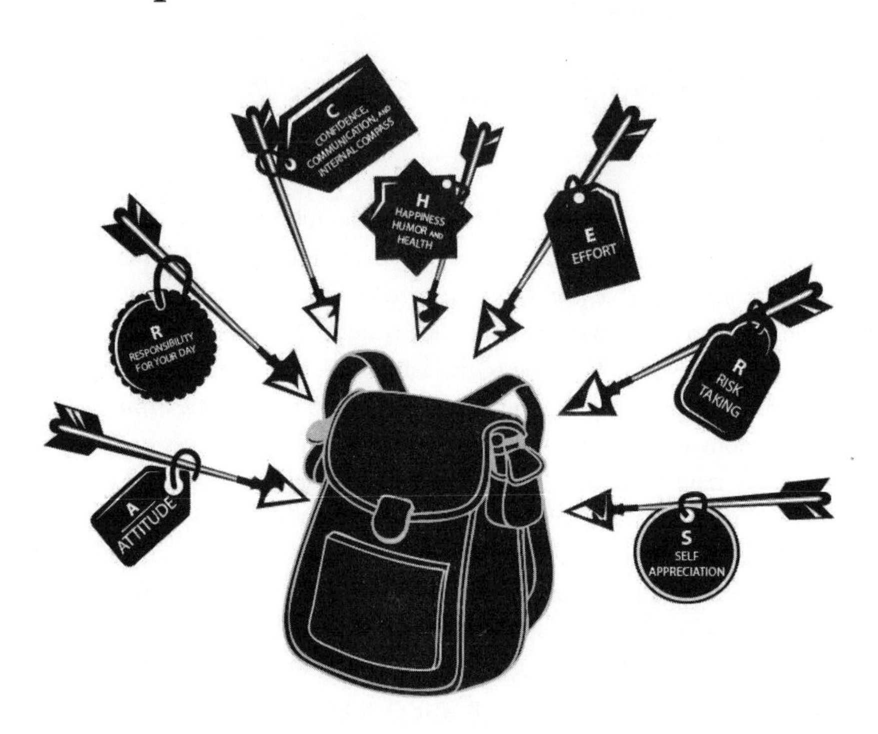

A—Attitude and learning from our mistakes

An optimistic attitude and a belief in a silver lining are important ingredients in securing resilience. People who are optimistic explain good events in terms of long-lasting causes. They believe they can overcome setbacks because they try to not focus on the negative. They focus more strongly on ways to make things work. We all have read stories similar to the "Little Engine that Could" or the train from *Dumbo* named Casey Jr. who kept on using the mantra "I think I can." Just saying "I think I can" may be the impetus for making a positive change.

People who are optimistic learn to appreciate that experienced failures are events, not people. Our children need to comprehend that throughout their lives, there will always be situations where they will make mistakes. People who are resilient review outcomes and put them in perspective (hopefully with an optimistic twist). We all need to expect that we cannot always do things perfectly or be the best all of the time. We need to help our children learn from their mistakes and turn them into lessons. For example, Jose elected not to practice as much as he needed to make the basketball team.

Rather than sulk in sorrow because he didn't make the team, he decided not to give up and spent an entire six months practicing the fundamentals. The next season he showed the coach he had what he needed to be a team member.

Let's take a look at two other examples of children and how they handled the outcome. The first scenario focuses on a young boy who is eleven and believes he has to be the best. Unfortunately, when he makes any mistakes, he takes them to heart and quickly disintegrates emotionally.

Emotional negativity seems to have an impact on his coping mechanisms. He tends to put up his armor and his actions are counterproductive. On the other hand, when Suzanne, who is also eleven, makes a mistake, she looks at it realistically and reflects on it. It's okay to make mistakes, especially when we can learn from them. Children must be willing to accept that their lives will be built on both successes and failures.

It's crucial to help children put these events in perspective. Perspective-taking is an approach to handling failure that could impact future resilience. As parents, our role could be to use situations of failure as teachable moments. Rather than focusing on negative outcomes, we should help our children realize that each outcome lends itself to new opportunities and new avenues to secure successes.

The cliché "turn your lemons into lemonade" is definitely appropriate. Children can take the lemons they have stumbled upon and use them in their recipe for life successes. When children begin to realize that it's okay to make mistakes, they will begin not to fear failing.

R—Responsible for your day

We need to teach our children that from the earliest of years they must learn to become responsible for who they are and their lives in general. The belief that *I am responsible for my day* needs to be a precept that our children see and live by on a daily basis. How many of us have witnessed our children, or even ourselves, making excuses for something that occurs? It's okay to be honest and take responsibility for things that have not worked out. By doing so, children begin to realize that they need to be accountable and must take responsibility. We take responsibilities not only for favorable outcomes but also for unfavorable outcomes. We suggest that teaching our children to accept accountability for their actions is critical.

Ultimately, if we can teach our children to live by the motto, *"I am responsible for my day,"* then they will be able to persevere and act with more confidence. They will also realize that, although they can rely on others to help pave their roads, the ultimate responsibility is theirs.

It's also equally important for children to realize that accepting responsibility requires honest appraisal and accountability of their efforts. Think of all of the examples that we can bring to the table. Rather than blaming your brother for not getting your room cleaned up, or blaming the dog for chewing up your homework, we need to help children take the responsibility for the actions they have selected. We all should follow the belief popularized by Nike—*Just Do It!*

Responsibility also pertains to developing a sense of strong morals and values. At the end of the day, having children who are morally responsible and concerned about others is a tremendous blessing. These young people will grow up being concerned about the welfare of others and they will become helpful. Children need to recognize that they are part of a world to which they are connected, and that they have a responsibility to give back. Therefore, being a caring individual who recognizes his or her commitment to social justice is a trait worth having. As McClain (2007) points out, children need to realize that the world is a better place because they're in it, and they can provide and contribute to the well-being of others.

When our children were younger, we had them volunteer as puppy raisers for guide dogs and work for the Special Olympics. Through these experiences, they learned that they could be givers rather than takers. They also became more sensitive to people that were down on their luck, and weren't as judgmental. Knowing that they could make a difference in people's lives was a powerful outcome.

Ultimately, children have to learn that they are responsible for their own day. They need to appreciate that if a change is needed, they have it within themselves to make things easier or harder on themselves. They have to accept their share of the responsibility.

C—Confidence, communication, and using your internal compass

A. Confidence

Confidence describes the feeling of knowing that we can handle a situation effectively and that we are not going to fall apart. We need to help children focus on individual strengths, rather than on perceived weaknesses. This isn't to say we don't encourage improvement, but in approaching our children we must facilitate positive change rather than defeatism.

We should not push children to take on more than they are realistically prepared to handle. When we give our children multiple tasks to work towards and they aren't capable, this may lead to perceived incompetence. We need to consider what to put on a child's plate to ascertain if our requests are reasonable.

The Zen proverb, "When the mind is ready, the teacher will come," makes a great deal of sense. By adjusting expectations that are reasonable, children will begin to recognize their skills and believe that they are capable. They have to have confidence in their abilities to tackle their weaknesses. It only makes sense. We are willing to gamble if we believe that we can win. Winners are those people who have learned through experience to do the uncomfortable things that losers won't do. A child's mindset has to be open to the new adventure; otherwise, he/she won't persevere. Carol Dweck, in her book *Mindset,* discusses this position and recognizes the importance of effort. She notes that people admire effort and it is that effort that "ignites that ability and turns it into accomplishment"(p. 41). All individuals, gifted athletes, and geniuses have to put out efforts to make a difference. Needless to say, focusing on flaws only weakens a response.

When talking to children about their confidence, we need to be honest about their achievements and be realistic, not deceitful. Over the years, we have had many parents come to us and discuss this issue. We have a simple response. Praise is good, but it must be realistic. When praise that isn't realistic is showered upon children, they begin to see through our half-truths. For example, telling children they are doing an excellent job when, in fact, they aren't, is unfair to those youngsters. It is like the parent who tells his young child that he is proud of him because he makes his bed, only to redo and tidy the bed when the child leaves. When returning, what is the message the child receives? My bed wasn't made well enough for you to leave it alone. On the other hand, we still can be supportive to our youngsters and use encouraging words during times that expectations are not met. Recognizing effort rather than the outcome can go a long way, especially when we are being truthful.

We also can help our children judge their performance. This goes hand in hand with metacognitive development where children, as they age, become more self-aware of how and why they think the way that they do. Helping children evaluate their abilities more realistically and gauge more accurately their accomplishments is a valuable tool. For example, Natalie is on a swim team and feels incompetent because she does not win the heats she is racing in. There are several options that can be drawn, including finding a swim competition where her skills are commensurate to the competition. On the other hand, we can also have her evaluate her performance against previous trials. If her times are improving, she is in fact doing better. That needs to be the element that we are focusing upon and should applaud.

B. Communication: Using positive self-talk

Children need to learn to use the language of optimism and apply positive self-talk rather than espousing negativity. It's a known fact that when children use excessive negativity in their language, it weakens their response to cope with setbacks. When a child says "I can't," it often means "I won't." As parents, it would be helpful to model and demonstrate the use of positive language in the child's everyday usage. In this manner, our children begin to recognize that being more positive and uplifting typically gets better responses from others. People who are often negative turn off others.

Sometimes, to demonstrate the power of self-talk, we can apply this simple example known as kinesiology. Have a child put out his/her dominant arm and then tell him/her that he/she needs to strongly resist your push. We will repeat the exercise twice. In the first scenario, we ask the child to say in a low voice (while resisting you pushing down on their arm) *I am a weak person,* or *a bad person.* This goes on for about five seconds. The exercise is repeated, but, in the next example the child is asked to use an affirming quote such as *I am strong* or *I am invincible.* What is typically noticed is that when the child uses positive self-talk the arm remains higher. We need to spend the time to teach our children to apply the language of optimism rather than defeatism.

C. Utilizing your internal compass

Being a comeback kid means that you need to find your way both in times of supreme joy as well as in times of adversity. Resilience must include your ability to get to where you need to go, even if life throws you detours. When life's routes change, as inevitably happens, you need to consult your internal compass to maintain alignment with your acknowledged route. Our compass begins to function as soon as we are able to reason and make personal choices and will continue to operate until the day we close our eyes for the last time.

The Chinese long ago (approximately 2,200 years) invented the compass to guide us along our chosen paths. People fortunately possess an internal compass which, in a similar fashion, allows us to remain aligned and true with our chosen routes in life. The possibility of losing one's route (and acknowledging that fact) is a concern that parents wish to convey to their children—hence the need to consult periodically one's internal compass. As parents, our role needs to be to help our child activate his/her compass or GPS and to help the child realize its value.

H—Happiness and a way of thinking: Practicing optimism and good health

The backpack wouldn't be complete unless it was sprinkled and spiked with happiness, a good sense of humor, and a healthy body. These three variables (as discussed earlier) are synergistic in creating a perception of optimism. We believe that all these factors promote life satisfaction and resilience and open us to confronting life's challenges. A healthy body and a happy mind help us to make the best of life. Although happiness may be dependent on many variables, including our temperament and life's fortunes or misfortunes, a great deal of perceived happiness is dependent on our choice to find that silver lining and to be content. As parents, we should model happiness and help our children realize that happiness is within their grasp. All they have to do is look for and find safe and healthy choices that make them content. Many entities can enhance our child's happiness, including finding enjoyment through humor, a positive mindset, success, faith, exercise, and friendships. Jeremy Bentham in 1830 said, "Create all the happiness you are able to create, remove all the misery you are able to remove." Happiness is the hallmark of well-being and is the glue that promotes satisfaction in life. Happiness also includes helping children find inner peace. Our backpack is more vibrant when packed with this magical elixir.

When children allow others to make them feel inferior, it only damages their sense of well-being and demotes in their minds that they are capable and lovable people. To be buoyant in our lives, we need to become our greatest advocate rather than our utmost enemy. Eleanor Roosevelt said, "Nobody can make you feel inferior without your consent." We need to endorse that belief and help our children live by this motto.

It is essential that all children learn positive coping mechanisms to deal with failure or negative feedback from others. They could also benefit from some stress reduction techniques. Dean Ornish (1990), who is the director of the Preventive Medicine Research Institute in California, believes that we can reduce disease with programs that include stress management, diet, and exercise. Children who are highly stressed are at risk for numerous psychosocial disorders. We strongly endorse that all children learn to apply techniques of guided imagery and relaxation. Learning techniques to relax one's breathing (including yoga) can also be a way to suppress stressful situations. There are numerous resources that can be found online or at local bookstores that can teach children strategies for stress reduction. These alternatives will help bring the mind-body-spirit into harmony. In essence, reducing perceived stress, changing a mindset from awfulness to awesomeness, and coping with disappointments are all ingredients to promoting resiliency.

E—Effort: It is important to try

When thinking of avoiding situations, we may often envision an ostrich burying its head into the sand. Our children need to realize they can't run away from their problems. It's important to try and that the effort makes a difference. We should acknowledge our children's effort and become more encouraging.

R—Risk-taking

Being a risk-taker is a critical element in our suggested backpack. Children need to become risk-takers and to view their lives symbolically as being full glasses, rather than half-full or empty. When we think about it, the only way to grow in life is to take risks and to get involved. Taking chances allows us to move forward, even if we may stumble. The effort of moving on is worthwhile. Where would we be today without risk-takers who tried to change the world and weren't afraid of some of the detours to get there?

Becoming a risk-taker is a valuable attribute in our backpack of resilience. Taking chances leads to new opportunities. Some risks may not work out, but hopefully, many will. André Gide, the French novelist who won the Nobel Prize for literature in 1947, stated, *"You cannot discover new oceans unless you have the courage to leave the shore."* We need to reinforce our children's willingness to secure new ways of learning and doing. Like others who have tried, when they are willing to leave their secure shores and seek alternative ways of doing things, they will continue to grow.

It's important for our children to recognize that anyone can handle positive outcomes, but it takes a stronger person to overcome challenges. Children must internalize the concept that you can't control the winds in life, but you can alter your sails so you continue to move forward. This is a tremendous lesson for our children to live by. Our children need to realize that life is filled not only with a wealth of positive outcomes, but also with misfortunes that will alter our route. Knowing that you can handle things and do the best you can is a gift that we need to be sure to place into that backpack. Children who are more capable of realizing they can handle things when they go wrong (because over time this will indeed happen) are children that will be more successful in navigating through their journey of life.

S—Self-Appreciation: Like yourself

All children come in different sizes, shapes, and abilities. Recognizing this allows our children to learn to judge themselves realistically rather than constantly comparing themselves to others.

A child who is resilient believes the mantra, "I am a capable and lovable person who deserves good things." Although self-appreciation is the last element to be packed into the backpack, it is probably the most important variable to have along. You have to believe in yourself and like who you are to proceed on your journey. Author Alvin Price was quoted as saying, "Parents need to fill a child's bucket of self-esteem so high that the rest of the world cannot poke enough holes to drain it dry." Throughout our children's early years, it must be our goal to help our children find their assets rather than dwell on their weaknesses. We can help them by acting as treasure hunters, attempting to unearth their riches for the world and them to see. When discovering these treasures, we help our children capture their hearts and souls by highlighting their riches. It is amazing that some gems are so tarnished that their worth is unseen and devalued. Helping children polish who they are allows them to begin to recognize their unique assets. All children must appreciate that they need to be their own best friends.

Final Thoughts

As our Parent-Child Dance treatise is about to end, with what other words of wisdom can we leave you? About a year ago we met a young man who had been married for about two years. While talking with us, he noted that his wife was ready to start a family. He, on the other hand, wasn't as keen and noted he was in the negotiating phase. A few months later, he conceded that he had lost that battle and was anxiously awaiting the birth of their child. Over the period of the pregnancy, we met on a couple of occasions and he admitted being afraid and excited at the same time. A month ago his son

Cruz was born, and he hasn't stopped smiling since. He was a bit weathered from not sleeping as much, but excited about his new voyage in life. How many of us remember those moments?

We believe that the Parent-Child Dance metaphor is a wonderful way to capture our interactions with our children. Parenting is about our movements with our children, and how we plan our steps to support their growth. Parenting, like choreography, is about the process that helps us experience and live the moments. Sure, parenting will be rich with memories of golden grand times, but there will be moments where we will pull out our hair in total desperation. That is what makes parenting so phenomenal. We don't always know where the road will lead us.

Although we want to love our children, we often have told parents that they don't have to be their child's best friend. We want our children to love and respect us, but there will be times that we have to make unpopular decisions in their upbringing. Perhaps they will be unpopular for the moment, but over time hopefully many of these decisions will help us bring up our children to become happy and self-sufficient adults.

Throughout this manuscript we have explored not only a wealth of dance moves (choreography of parenting), but also some of the unique dynamics and issues that we will experience with our children over the years (teenage years, friendship, resilience, etc.). The most critical message that we want to impart is the recognition that parenting is such a tremendous opportunity for all of us. Don't miss the window of opportunity and fear what the outcome will be, but rather cherish and commit going on the journey. For some of us, we dream about our chance of becoming a parent and for our opportunity "to do it right." For most, the years of active parenting will be the best experiences of their lives. (It never really ends. We will still be parents to our adult children.) In parenthood, we have the chance to mold a human and prepare that child for the future.

At parenting meetings, there are often occasions where parents pour their hearts out. Most of the comments are filled with rich sentimental memories of times gone by too quickly. Parents dwell on the good times and can articulate with great accuracy memories that make them smile or drip tears. There are also parents who open their hearts about disappointing years that have left them feeling unfulfilled. We don't have all the answers to their comments and questions, nor should we be expected to. We do know that when you have the opportunity to actively parent, you need to embrace that role and not lose that window of time. We believe that our dance with our children will have numerous twists and turns, but to accomplish our ultimate aspirations (for our children) we must sprinkle our love and devotion with parenting methods that will help our children grow. We have highlighted many of these strategies that should make your dance more meaningful and impacting to you and your child. You cannot be passive in accepting the responsibilities of bringing up children. It is important to respond proactively with your love and concern. As we close, we are reminded of noted psychologist and writer Wayne Dyer's quotation: "When you dance, your purpose is not to get to a certain place on the floor. It's to enjoy each step along the way." Dance and celebrate your budding relationship with your children. You will be able to personally experience the magnificence of the sunrises and the sunsets of raising your children.

References

American Psychological Association. (2014). *The road to resilience.* Washington, DC. Retrieved from http://www.apa.org/helpcenter/road-resilience.aspx

Association for Psychological Science. (2010, March 24). Optimism boosts the immune system. *Science Daily.* Retrieved from www.sciencedaily.com/releases/2010/03/100323121757.htm

Brooks, R. & Goldstein, S. (2001). *Raising resilient children: Fostering strength, hope and optimism in your children.* Chicago: Contemporary Books.

Dweck, C. (2006). *Mindset: The new psychology of success.* New York: Ballentine Books.

Frankl. V. E. (2006). *Man's Search for Meaning.* Boston, MA: Beacon Press.

Ginsburg, K. R. & Jablow, M. M. (2011). *Building resilience in children and teens: Giving kids roots and wings.* Elk Grove Village, IL: American Academy of Pediatrics.

McClain, B. (2007, Winter). Building resilience in children. *Healthy Children Magazine.* Retrieved from http://www.healthychildren.org/Documents/Healthy-Children-Magazine/HealthyChildren-07Winter.pdf

Ornish, D. (1990). *Dr. Dean Ornish's program for reversing heart disease.* New York: Random House.

Perry, B. D. (2006, April). Resilience: Where does it come from? *Scholastic Early Childhood Today.* Retrieved from http://www.scholastic.com/browse/article.jsp?id=3746847

Seligman, M. (2006). *Learned Optimism: How to Change Your Life and Your Mind.* New York: Vintage Books.

Timbs, J. (1825) The three Rs – Reading Writing and Rithmetic: Speech by Sir William Curtis (1795) at a school dinner. *The Mirror of Literature, Amusement and Instruction,* Volume 5, p. 75. London: J. Limbird.